What readers say about The 5:2 Diet Book:

The author has been there and done it, and so it's like your best friend sharing her tips with you. I've already seen some great results.

Kate's honest & easy to read guide helped me through the first fast day. When I felt wobbly I read the book! I loved the chatty way she takes you through shares her journey. If you are contemplating the 5:2, this should be your bible.

Being a reasonably fit, sporty male, I was as interested in the long-term health benefits as the potential weight loss. Kate Harrison's book is written in an extremely readable style, the science is explained in a non-baffling way, and it's full of motivational tips and examples (as well as ideas for low-calorie menus/dishes that you don't need to be Jamie Oliver to prepare). Inspirational reading!

Worth every penny to help change your attitude to food and be healthier.

This book doesn't promise miracles, doesn't sell the reader expensive supplements, nor does it over-complicate matters. It keeps the concept simple, straight forward, easy to apply, and flexible. Just like the dietary approach.

With Kate's help, I survived the fast days. I have heard so many success stories so keeping my fingers crossed but as it promises health benefits too, it can't be wrong!

All reviews for the Kindle edition

Safety Note

I've put together this guide because this way of eating has made such a big difference to me and I wanted to share my experiences and those of others who are making this work. But this ebook is written for information only and is not intended as medical advice, or as a substitute for medical advice, diagnosis or treatment. I have also included links for information and interest but have no control over their contents.

Always consult a doctor before making dietary changes, particularly if you have any pre-existing conditions. Neither the author nor publisher or associates can be held responsible for any loss or claim resulting from the use or misuse of information and suggestions contained in this book, or for the failure to take medical advice.

Finally, never disregard professional medical advice or delay medical treatment because of something you have read in this book.

Copyright © 2012 Kate Harrison

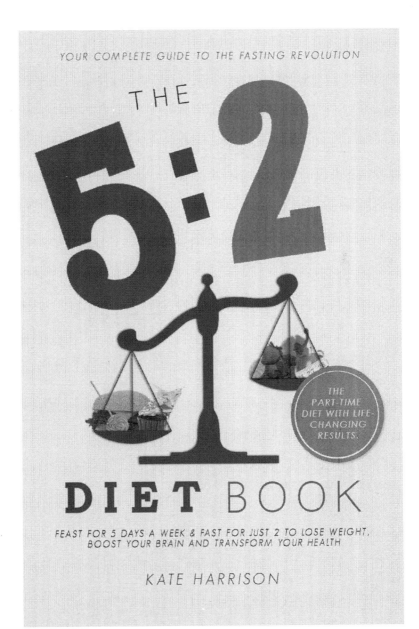

YOUR COMPLETE GUIDE TO THE FASTING REVOLUTION

THE 5:2

THE PART-TIME DIET WITH LIFE-CHANGING RESULTS.

DIET BOOK

FEAST FOR 5 DAYS A WEEK & FAST FOR JUST 2 TO LOSE WEIGHT,
BOOST YOUR BRAIN AND TRANSFORM YOUR HEALTH

KATE HARRISON

Why reading this book will revolutionise your body and your future

Imagine a diet that lets you eat the foods you love, most of the time.

That enables you to lose weight steadily.

That could reduce your risk of cancer, heart disease, diabetes and Alzheimer's.

That makes your brain sharper and your body more efficient.

That changes your attitude to hunger and food forever.

A diet that involves no special 'low-cal' or 'lite' foods and will probably save you money.

That's completely flexible, to fit your lifestyle.

That suits men and women, those new to diets and those who've tried everything.

A diet you'll want to stick with for life.

Stop Imagining. The 5:2 Diet is real.

November 2012
Dear Reader,

Four months ago, I watched a TV programme that changed my life.

I almost didn't write that line, because it sounds so cheesy, but it happens to be true. Sixty minutes of viewing set the scene for a huge change in my attitude to dieting, introduced me to an exciting new branch of medical science – and gave me the tools to begin transforming my body.

Of course, I've had to do the hard work myself, but the programme opened the door to the world of intermittent fasting and calorie restriction – the official name for an approach to health and diet which is gaining huge numbers of followers around the world. Many of them share their experiences for this book – experiences that are likely to inspire you to follow their lead!

What I've learned has made me feel in control of food, not the other way round. It's given me new hope that I can do something constructive to reduce my chances of developing cancer, dementia and diabetes, which have had devastating effects on members of my family. It's a lifestyle I want to follow... well, for life. The rapid popularity of this approach is typical of many hyped diets. You know the ones. They're flavour of the month, and then they drop out of fashion almost as quickly.

But intermittent fasting is one diet craze that is anything BUT crazy

It's sustainable, adaptable and it might help you live longer. It's also very simple, and the 'fasting' part isn't nearly as punishing as it sounds because - whisper it – you never have to have to go a day without eating. You simply work one, two or more days of low-calorie eating into your weekly routine, and forget all about 'dieting' the rest of the time. Until you step on the scales...

And it's not just about how you look or how much you weigh - it's also about how your body works, right down to cellular level

Reducing your calorie intake radically for short periods, triggers changes in your body's metabolism and brain function that can cut the risk of the diseases we all fear: cancer, heart disease, Alzheimer's and diabetes. There are benefits for your body and your brain as your body works hard to repair cells damaged by lifestyle and ageing.

You might well look younger – and you'll definitely feel it!

This lifestyle will also change your attitude to food and eating for the better.

The benefits of fasting have been known in medical circles for some time, but finally this way of eating is going mainstream.

There are no hidden gimmicks, no complications, no over-priced supplements or revolting meal replacements. In fact, this way of eating will save you money.

Definitely not just for girls...

This is a diet that both men and women are adopting whole-heartedly, because it's so flexible and fuss-free. Fast Days offer a 'mini break' from worrying about food – and because you only have to stick to any kind of plan for a couple of days a week, you don't feel deprived. Plus, research suggests dieters don't overcompensate on the 'Feast' days but adopt healthier habits without even thinking or noticing.

**The ultimate practical guide to the most
sustainable diet there is**

The 5:2 Diet Book has all the information you need to
start tomorrow. Or - if you're reading this before
breakfast - you could even start today!

The book takes you step-by-step through embracing a
lifestyle that suits your needs and goals. There is no
proscriptive list of dos and don'ts, no list of 'Banned' or
'Sinful' foods. You work out the maximum number of
calories you can eat on your Fast Days - then stick to that
limit for a couple of days a week (or once a week, or every
other day - it depends what suits you and how much
weight, if any, you want to lose). Then you eat normally
the rest of the time.

If it's that simple, why do I need a book about it?

Well, maybe you don't - if you stick to 500 calories a day
(if you're a woman) or 600 (if you're a man) on your 'fast'
days, then you'll almost certainly benefit.

But, when I started following this regime, I did have lots
of questions and uncertainties and I looked in vain for a
guide that would help me find the right approach.

Why I've written this book

Once I'd distilled all the information I could find, for my own use, I decided it would make sense to put it together and create the consumer guide I couldn't find... so here it is.

It'll be your companion when you start, with lots of practical information, recipes, meal plans and encouragement to help you launch this way of life and alter your body and approach to food for good. Pretty soon, this way of life should feel like second-nature - but the case studies and the remarkable scientific research underpinning this diet should help keep you on track. I've spoken to dozens of other 5:2 dieters, male and female, of all ages, who share their wisdom, successes and excitement about the changes they've seen.

I'm no doctor. I'm just a failed dieter who happens to have found something that works for me, at last. And I am pretty certain it can work for you too. I happen to be a vegetarian and a 'Great British Bake Off' addict, but whether you're a dedicated foodie, or not fussed about cooking . . . a cuddly carnivore or a gluttonous veggie . . . a carb-lover or a party animal, you can make this fit your life.

Health Warning

I have no medical training, though I've always taken a keen interest in food and nutrition. I'm going to share my experiences, and those of other successful 5:2 dieters.

But there are people who shouldn't follow this diet: children and teenagers; pregnant women; people with compromised immunity, diabetes, metabolic syndrome or adrenal imbalances.

In addition, anyone with a history of eating disorders should definitely not undertake this without talking to their doctors.

In fact, even if you are otherwise healthy, talk to your GP - they're on your side, and if you are committed to losing weight, it'll make their job easier! It's also quite likely they'll know all about 5:2 – many doctors are trying it for themselves!

How this book works

The 5:2 Diet Book has three parts. Part One explains the thinking behind the diet - including medical and psychological research about why losing weight this way can boost your body in some incredible ways. These chapters alternate with my own diary, where I share highs and lows I encountered as I adapted to this new way of thinking about food and diet.

Part Two contains all the practical information you need to make 5:2, 6:1 or Alternate Day Fasting (ADF) work for you. I've included information on how to prepare for the Fast Days and how to stay motivated, plus guidance on exercise and calorie counting, along with loads of real-life success stories and experiences to keep you on track.

Part Three focuses on food ideas for your Fast Days, with lots of simple options for meals and snacks to appeal to all tastes, including suggestions for seasonal eating and sample menus to stop you feeling hungry. Finally, I've included a resources section for further reading though there are also links throughout the text to interesting articles on the internet that offer more information on particular topics. I've abbreviated the links to make them easier to type into your browser if you want to find out more by going online! Alternatively, you can download a single list of links free of charge via my website: go to kate-harrison.com/5-2diet

Can't cook, won't cook? Not a problem!

I know preparing food when you're on a diet can be a chore, so there are also ideas from 5:2 fans who've suggested their favourite ready-made meals. Many of us prefer to leave cooking till 'Feast' days when you're free to make the dishes you love!

The simplest, most grown-up diet in the world

This diet – and this book - treats you like an adult. Pick and choose what makes sense to you. A lot of the science is new and evolving, so there are some questions which don't yet have definitive answers. My job is to offer you all the options so that, like me, you can find your own personalised way of working intermittent fasting into your life.

But have no doubt - this is working for me and thousands more of us. Word of the diet has spread far and wide - because it works. And it could work for you too.

Of course, I love feeling slimmer, but this is about much more than vanity. Like most of us, I know that there are many diseases like cancer and diabetes that have blighted my family - now at last I feel I can try something practical to improve my odds.

This book isn't about rules. It's about freedom. What's stopping you?

Kate Harrison, November 2012

Contents

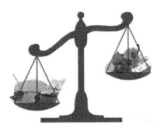

Part One: The 5:2 Revolution

What the diet does, how it works, why it's for you

Chapter One: Living the 5:2 Way: feast, fast and be happy!

I am on a diet. But this one is different.

No, really. I understand your scepticism. I've spent almost two-thirds of my life on a diet. And ninety-nine per cent of my *adult* life either dieting or feeling rubbish about how I look.

I'm not unusual. Most women I know – and increasing numbers of men – have a love/hate relationship with their bodies and with food. OK, we can blame Size Zero actresses for giving us unrealistic expectations about how we should look (and sending us to the biscuit tin for comfort). Or we could pin it on multi-national food companies or takeaway joints for trying to get us to eat more, more, MORE!

But short of never watching a movie and growing all your food from scratch, there's little we can do about the external causes of what the press call the Obesity Epidemic.

What we *can* do is find a way of eating that works for us.

And – to my astonishment – I think I might have done that at last, at the ripe old age of forty-four.

For me – and many others you'll hear from in this book – it's *revolutionary.*

What this diet is like

For breakfast this morning, I savoured a chocolate and almond croissant from the best bakery I know, the one that's tormented me with its forbidden treats since I moved into a house approximately thirty-five steps from its doors.

But it doesn't torment me anymore. Because thanks to the 5:2 Diet, I know I can indulge - even, occasionally, over-indulge - but still lose weight.

Tomorrow I'll be fasting, one of two Fast Days a week (the 2 in 5:2) when I make a big change. Strictly speaking, this isn't a true fast, because I can eat up to three small meals - but most 5:2 dieters do call these reduced calorie days Fast Days.

I will eat roughly 25% of the calories my body actually needs: at that level, the way my metabolism works will change, but I won't feel faint or unbearably hungry, as I probably would with a 'true' fast.

I'll eat at lunchtime and dinner time: as it's winter, I'll probably have a soup for lunch, and a vegetable curry side dish for dinner, with some extra veg and perhaps a yogurt or a piece of fruit for pudding.

Yes, it *is* limited - but I don't care because the day after, I can forget counting calories and eat the things I enjoy.

Suddenly, food is all not about the Forbidden. I'm enjoying a balanced diet without feeling guilty about sharing a bottle of really delicious red wine, or having a full English for Sunday brunch.

So long as I keep a close eye on my eating habits for two days a week, I know I can enjoy a little of what I fancy the rest of the time – and still lose weight.

Since I discovered this way of eating three months ago I've lost over a stone (16lbs or 7.25 kg), without cutting out any of the foods I love: cheese, chocolate, the odd cocktail (make mine a Mojito). I haven't gone crazy - I probably have shifted to a more balanced diet on my five 'normal' days, but without making conscious changes. I simply have a much greater awareness of what my body needs, and when. I eat when I'm hungry and without bingeing.

And I savour my food.

Don't just take my word for it...

I've surveyed dozens of dieters who are changing their lives for good.

Dieters like software architect Andrew, and his five workmates, who all decided to begin the diet at the same time. Like many men, none had followed 'named' diets before, but were inspired by the simplicity and science of this approach. They've been tracking their progress over the last nine weeks:

We all starting losing weight at different times. I lost a lot of weight immediately, but slowed down later on. Overall we have lost about the same, around four kilograms and our weight losses week on week appear to be stabilising. The point of the 5:2 diet is not really about losing weight, it's about health. The improvement in blood pressure, cholesterol etc. is why we are doing it.

Andrew, 42

Four kilograms is almost nine pounds – an impressive loss. But how are they finding it? Thirty-four-year-old Sunil went in with a very clear target:

My main motivation is to reduce my cholesterol - I'm a British Indian, so live mostly on an Indian diet which isn't the best for reducing cholesterol. I wanted to try a diet that doesn't have a major impact on my life and this fits the bill. It's so easy. The first week or two are not hard, but it just takes a little discipline. I now don't even think about hunger on starving days.

It feels normal. I find that my general appetite is less throughout the week - I used to have the urge to binge in evenings after dinner I've lost 3.2 kilograms and added an extra notch to my belt. I'm getting my cholesterol tested soon.

Forty-one-year-old software engineer Kostas has always been athletic, but has still struggled with blood pressure and weight concerns. Until now.

I've lost 2 kilos, feel much better (psychologically), less bloated so I fit better in my clothes. The diet works, and there are hundreds of meals you can plan during a fasting day. The diet is keeping us healthier without depriving us of anything. Eventually, it will become a way of life. Now, even during my non-fasting days I am aware of what I eat and how much. I don't feel that I restrict myself from any kind of food that I like, because I can tell myself that I can eat it in my non-fasting days. My fasting days feel like I am cleansing myself.

The freedom – and the cost savings – appeal to Myfanwy, who has lost a pound a week and is also showing a welcome reduction on blood pressure:

I can fit it around my life - work, teenage children, meals out, celebrations. It costs me nothing - and saves me money (no lunches or snacks on fasting days). There's no complicated calorie balancing and no inevitable guilt when one cannot keep a diet up day after miserable day.

Myfanwy, 49

Dieters of all ages and lifestyles are finding the results incredibly rewarding.

It's simple, and it works! I've lost over a stone in three months. Clothes fit again. Belly has gone. Huzzah! OK I get a tad hungry sometimes, but nothing that reduces me to tears..

John, 58

Kirsty has lost eleven pounds in twelve weeks.

It has taken me to a BMI of about 22 or 23. I noticed a change in body shape and I like the "part time" nature of the diet best - the Fast Days are restrictive (but they've never

21

driven me absolutely mad) and I always keep to the fast because I know that I can eat what I want the next day. Obviously the weight loss has been pleasing and has made the diet worth continuing with. I have actually enjoyed feeling my tummy rumble as I realised that it rarely does ordinarily! After four days of eating normally, I actually look forward to feeling cleansed by a Fast Day!

Kirsty, 38

The flexibility of the approach means people are trying out different variations – several of the men I've surveyed have gone for a stricter fast, for simplicity and speed:

I have had limited success with restricted calorie diets in the past, but was unable to keep up with them as a lifestyle. In under four weeks I've lost lots of weight and 2 inches off my waist. I love it! No calorie counting makes it much more sustainable for me. I believe it's much easier to water fast on fasting days than to consume the 500-600 cals that some do.

Rob, 42

The Healthiest Diet?

So far, so good. We're losing weight and inches, and feeling motivated.

But there are other, even more important reasons why many of us have decided to do this diet:

My mother had every illness under the sun and I don't want to follow in her footsteps. I have a young family and wish to be around, plus the weight loss and memory improvements would be a bonus. I've already lost two stone and inches from the stomach (which would suggest a reduction in the risk of heart disease). Plus, no saggy skin and my boobs have stayed the same size, even though they're usually the first to go on a diet!

Fiona, 41

I wanted to lower my blood pressure and cholesterol and after two months, so far, so good. It's easy and the more you do it, the easier it gets. I like that it makes scientific sense.

Paul, 47

I'm doing this for weight loss and for health reasons. My father has Alzheimer's, plus I have high blood pressure.

Sarah, 49

Like Fiona and Sarah, I have concerns about my family's medical history, particularly with regard to metabolic disorders like diabetes and cancer. Every year, I have a mammogram even though I'm not old enough to 'qualify' for one in the UK yet. That's because of my family history. I had my annual check this week – a stark reminder of the breast cancer diagnoses that have hit my mother, aunt, grandmother and many other female relatives.

But what I've learned has given me fresh hope. Research is going on right now with women of my age at higher risk of breast cancer – they are following a 5:2 style diet and the early signs are very encouraging. Not only are they losing weight – in itself an effective tool in reducing cancer risk – but tests are also revealing genetic changes which could help protect them from the disease they fear most.

The work is also suggesting improvements in the body's response to insulin – which also feels incredibly relevant to me as I am at very high risk of developing Type II diabetes, with all the complications that ensue.

You will have your own concerns and genetic inheritance but it's almost certain that 5:2 will address some of them. So many of the conditions that scare us are on the 5:2 hit list because of the changes it makes to your body – see Chapters Three and Four for much more on the medical research.

The Diet that succeeds where others have failed?

The diet works brilliantly for all adults, but anecdotally, it seems it's proving especially popular among those aged 35+. It is around this age that we often begin to find it incredibly tough to shift weight, and also become more aware of our own mortality or of family tendencies towards developing chronic or life-threatening medical conditions.

> *Couldn't fit in my clothes, saw my photos at my brother's 50th (awful), where we're all overweight, worried about joints etc, scared of being disabled through fatness, felt that this offered an intelligent approach. Mum is losing her short term memory and if fasting staves that off, I will give it a whirl. I need my brain. Feel a bit more hopeful of avoiding some of the health issues affecting my parents (and my grandparents before they passed away).*
>
> *Linda, 52*

A Facebook group I set up (The 5:2 Diet – you're very welcome to join us) is full of motivating stories from men and women of all ages and occupations - and they're reporting the same great results. Not just weight loss, but also a feeling that you're doing something positive for your body.

Because the 5:2 diet has a huge advantage over other diets – it brings about physiological changes that help the body – and even the brain - heal itself.

Fasting does put stress on our systems but the way we respond to that stress seems overwhelmingly positive. Research in humans and animals shows that fasting tends to lower the amount of the IGF-1 hormone which plays a role in the development of cancer. It can also reduce blood pressure and cholesterol levels, activate processes that repair the body's cells, *and* even encourage the production of more neurons in the brain.

These effects are, of course, harder to measure on an individual basis than weight loss – but increasingly evidence suggests this way of eating has positive effects that far exceed the benefits of weight reduction alone.

I've gone into the medical research and the science in Chapter Three – it makes fascinating *and* motivating reading.

Back in Control

There's another benefit that didn't feature in the BBC programme, but has transformed the attitudes of many 5:2 dieters.

This year, I'd more or less resigned myself to being fat and frumpy forever. I felt out of control, and very depressed about my lack of willpower – yet I couldn't seem to find a way to overcome that.

To my surprise, my Fast Days have had a profound effect on the way I think and behave, and not only when I'm restricting calories. The experience of reconnecting with my appetite, and re-learning how to deal with occasional hunger pangs, has helped me and many other people get back in touch with how our bodies work.

I find fasting days very 'cleansing'. It has also made me realise that I can survive on a lot less calories than I thought I could. And periods of excess, e.g. Holidays, Christmas etc. can be 'put right' relatively effortlessly.

Claire, 43

Working really well for me. I like the discipline on two days (and the self-awareness of slight hunger discomfort), combined with complete freedom the rest of the week.

James, 43

I now think that all those diets promising 'you'll never feel hungry' have done us a disservice. Knowing the difference between eating because you need to, and eating because you are bored/thirsty/fed up is a basic skill, and one that can help you control and understand your weight issues.

It's bloody easy, and it's good to feel hungry. From years of dieting lore that advocated eating little and often, it feels like a relief to be able to skip meals and breakfast particularly.

Julia, 50

In Chapter Four, I delve deeper into the psychology of this lifestyle change.

The Simplest Diet

The simplicity of this diet is what makes it so irresistible to many of us. You decide how many days a week to monitor calories – and then either do some simple maths to work out your 'limit' or go for the average of 500 for women and 600 for men.

Then - you start. The foods you need on Fast Days can almost certainly be found in your cupboard, freezer, or definitely in your local supermarket. There's nothing specialised, no meal replacements to be bought or sent off for at huge expense.

> *I'm lazy when it comes to cooking so I keep things very simple – beans on toast for lunch and shop-bought soup for dinner. I won't be winning 'Masterchef' but I don't care because keeping it fuss-free is really important in staying on this diet.*
>
> *Katy, 30*

The only two tools that come in useful are a set of kitchen scales and either a calorie book or access to the internet or a smartphone so you can use online tools or apps to calculate your intake. But even those aren't compulsory.

> *I tend to stick to Birds Eye chicken or beef dinners, or variations on that theme. They're all weighed out and have the calories on the boxes, so it saves weighing things and calculating calories.*
>
> *Sally, 49*

If you follow the ready-made food suggestions in the second half of this book, you'll be able to do the diet without extra calorie counting.

The Oldest Diet

Fasting is a part of almost all organised religions, suggesting that those faiths have long had an awareness of the benefits for mind *and* body of taking a break from eating, or alternatively eating very simply and frugally.

But you don't have to have any specific religious belief to follow the 5:2 diet - what you're doing is taking advantage of wisdom that we're now rediscovering.

Not for everyone?

As I said in the introduction, there are groups of people who should not make such major changes in eating patterns including pregnant women or nursing mothers, children and teenagers, diabetics, those with other medical conditions, and those who have a great deal of weight to lose. I do know some new mothers and morbidly obese people who are making this diet work, but it would be a very bad idea to begin without medical supervision.

The same applies to people with a history of eating disorders or psychological issues around food or appearance. For most of us, eating less on a couple of days a week is easy to adopt, but like any habit, it could be taken to extremes which could damage your mental or physical health. If you have any worries, please, *please* do talk to a specialist before considering the 5:2 or intermittent fasting approach.

Indeed, to be safe, it's a good idea to talk to your GP about this, or any other dietary change. Sally is doing this already:

> *I'd suggest involving your doctor/practice nurse and going to be weighed there regularly too. Tell them what diet you're doing and discuss any problems you might be having. That way they can keep an eye on you and a medical record of how the diet is affecting you. Most surgeries are set up to support weight loss, so you shouldn't have any problems getting an appointment to be weighed.*
>
> *Sally, 49*

I must admit I haven't gone down this route myself. I'd already been advised by my GP to lose weight and knew my basic health indicators – blood pressure, heart rate, fasting blood sugar – gave no particular cause for concern.

But I did know I could count on their support to track the weight loss if need be. I'm looking forward to my next check-up so I can be told officially that I am in better shape!

In Chapter Two, I'll be talking about the maths of weight loss and how they relate to the 5:2 approach.

But before that, with apologies to Bridget Jones, here's the first of my 5:2 Diary entries, starting on the date that changed everything for me: August 6 2012.

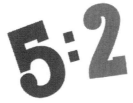

A Couch Potato Watches TV & Makes a
Decision

Weight 161 lbs/73 kg
Mood: guilty, resigned

Today I am the fattest I've ever been.

Even though I've started three diets
this year alone, I keep getting bigger. I
weigh eleven and a half stone (73 kg) - and
am only five foot four inches tall (when I
stand up *very* straight). So that gives me a
BMI of 27.6 - and anything 25 or above is
overweight. Eleven stone was bad enough - I
thought that would be my mental limit, the
moment where I took action, yet the weight
is still creeping on.

My size 14 jeans (which I always tend
to think of as a 16, as they're quite
generously cut) are slicing into my waist,
my bra is too tight and there are lumps and

bumps showing when I wear anything but the baggiest of tops. Worst of all, my belly is wobbly - I've always been curvy, with big hips and boobs, but my tummy is now catching up.

Has anyone seen my willpower?

This is the slippery slope. I feel out of control, frumpy, middle-aged and very, very cross with myself. I don't want to be gaining half a stone a year, wearing a size 18 or more before I'm fifty, feeling ashamed to go on the beach because I look like the fat lady on a seaside postcard.

Yet my willpower is diminishing with age, too. A few years ago, I managed to get to my lowest adult weight - a sylph-like eight and a half stone - thanks to low-carbing the vegetarian way. I felt good on it, wore skinny jeans for the first time, and really enjoyed eating lots of lovely cheese, Greek yogurt, nuts, berries and so on. And yet…

And yet even as people congratulated me on my success, a tiny part of me knew it couldn't last. I love bread, cakes and desserts. I have a huge recipe book collection and adore farmers' markets and nice restaurants, especially Indian or Italian places. Could I really turn my back on pasta, pilau rice and baked goodies for the rest of my life?

Plus, something didn't feel quite right about eating such a restricted diet: cutting out one food group seemed wrong. Sure enough, the weight crept back on. I tried low-carbing again this last month, but I couldn't convince myself it was something that would last. Because, frankly, it won't.

Fat and fearful...

This is not simply about vanity anymore. Both my parents have Type 2 Diabetes - the kind that starts in later life - and I've seen the complications it causes, to vision, joints and the skin. Their diagnoses also mean my chances of getting it are very high.

Plus, there's the strong family

history of breast cancer on Mum's side - and a friend who has recovered from breast cancer raised doubts about how reliant I was on dairy products on the low-carb veggie diet. Dairy is something she's minimised since she went into remission because she's concerned that too much of it might increase her cancer risk.

Though being overweight increases the risk of cancer, too. It's hard to know what to do for the best.

How much more desperate do I need to become?

I've joined a gym *again* and am trying to go, but, realistically, three cross-trainer sessions a week are going to burn 1,200 cals maximum. Apparently to lose a pound of fat, you have to cut 3,500 calories from your diet, or do 3,500-worth of activity without eating any extra food. Gym-going alone is not going to be enough. I've joined a site, MyFitnessPal.com, to monitor what I'm eating, but it's labour intensive and it doesn't include listings for the days I eat out, because it's impossible to know the calorie count of restaurant food.

Yesterday, I found myself Googling diet drugs - the kind that 'bind' to the fat you eat and help you pass it before it gets digested. The side-effects are utterly revolting and yet I went as far as filling in an online form to find out if I'd be eligible for them. I am, but apparently they're out of stock.

So I'm not alone in seeking a quick fix.

A Lost Cause...

Maybe I just have to accept this is the shape I'll stay. I could take down all the mirrors in the house to start with...

There's a TV programme I'm going to watch tonight about fasting - the description of the show is intriguing. But let's face it - I don't have the willpower to do a 'normal' diet, never mind a fast. I suspect it'll just give me even more to feel guilty about.

10.05pm

Wow.

That was an amazing programme… really fascinating, full of counter-intuitive science and new information - plus fasting REALLY worked for the presenter.

Even better, it wasn't a 'true' fast - he did still eat on his fasting days, just an awful lot less.

The potential benefits also seem to go way beyond weight loss. There's a possibility that 'intermittent calorie restriction' - a more accurate but less catchy description than fasting - could reduce the risk of breast cancer, diabetes, heart disease and even Alzheimer's.

This is a diet that could offer more than weight loss alone.

But I have been here before, with low-carb, high-fibre, tum/bum/thigh. The fact is, miracle diets don't exist.

Or do they?

Chapter Two: The maths of weight loss – and why Fasting adds up

Slim people don't just look better by the pool.

They also live longer. The *rats*.

It's the reason your doctor checks your weight and calculates your BMI - Body Mass Index – when you have a check-up. The BMI is a simple calculation based on your height and weight (some would say too simple: read Dr John Briffa's blog for an awful lot more about this: the link to type into your browser is bit.ly/TsfjeU or don't forget, I've created a free downloadable list of links to make it easier for readers of the print edition to read more: you can use straight from your computer at kate-harrison.com/5-2diet).

If your BMI is over 25 - or 23 for some ethnic groups - you're officially overweight. And if it's over 30, you're classed as obese: the higher the figure goes, the higher the statistical risk of disease.

You can either calculate it by this formula, or by using the chart over the page:

BMI = Weight (kg) / [Height (m) x Height (m)]

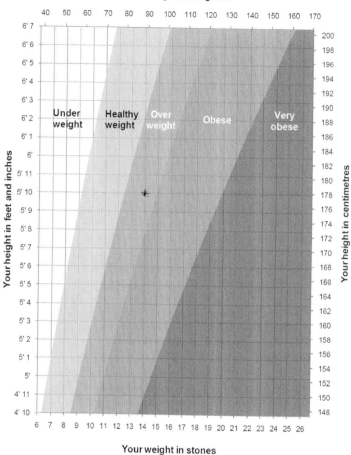

Your weight in kilograms

Your height in feet and inches

Your height in centimetres

Your weight in stones

Under weight | Healthy weight | Over weight | Obese | Very obese

As a measure, BMI isn't perfect – you may have heard about rugby players or athletes who train for hours a day yet are classed as 'obese' by BMI standards because they have lean bodies with high muscle mass. BMI is also pretty hopeless in children. Plus, the risk calculations are based on large-scale studies so it can't tell you much about YOUR personal specific risks, which depend on so many other factors: family history, genetics, lifestyle, environment.

Lies, damned lies – and home truths?

But before you write off the BMI, remember statistics don't *always* lie. For every chain-smoking Great Aunt Winifred, who was the size of a horse and ate like one, and celebrated her 100th birthday with a bottle of gin for breakfast, there are millions of us whose diets are damaging our health.

Excess weight can increase our risk of developing a range of diseases and conditions including:

☐ *High blood pressure*
☐ *Type 2 diabetes*
☐ *Coronary heart disease*
☐ *Strokes*
☐ *Gallbladder disease*
☐ *Cancer of the breast or colon*
☐ *Osteoarthritis*
☐ *Respiratory problems*

Of course, you could hope you're going to be the exception that proves the rule. Or you can try to maintain to a 'healthy' weight to keep the statistics on your side.

Whatever your BMI, the truth is you probably don't need a figure to tell you you've put on too much weight. My guess is that if you're reading this book then you, like me, want to reduce your risks of these life-shortening, or quality-of-life reducing, conditions.

As well as looking better by the pool...

But, as we all know, losing weight is easier said than done:

> *I've tried every diet going! I was first taken to a slimming club at the age of 11 and have been dieting ever since, sometimes with success, sometimes not. I originally lost weight when I was 17 by starving. I would have 1oz All Bran (dry) in the morning, an apple lunch time and plain salad in the evening. I used to tell my mum I was having lunch at college so that I didn't have to eat in the evening. I did this for 2 years and got down to 8 stone which is too thin for my 5 foot 7 inches! Once I started eating normally again the weight piled on. In my mid 20's I went to a Slimming Magazine slimming club and got to within 7lbs of my goal weight. Again, as soon as I started*

eating normally the weight piled on! Then Weight Watchers - Slimming World, Rosemary Conley classes! I've tried Atkins, Paul McKenna, Scarsdale ... far too many diets to mention!!!

Jeanny, 53

I've tried all sorts - from The Cabbage Soup diet, Slimfast and the Beyoncé diet to Weight Watchers. The one that's worked best for long term weight loss was WW. I've had two successes there, though gradually the weight has gone back on. I'm greedy, really, it's that simple.

Sarah 49

Eating too much makes you fat - and other annoying things thin people say

People who don't struggle with their weight often have a maddening habit of stating the obvious.

'Losing weight is easy,' they'll say. 'Couldn't be simpler. Eat less, move more.'

Or they might point out the basic maths - that if you consume more food (or calories) than you burn off, you'll put weight on, and if you do the opposite then you'll lose it.

'Oh, if I feel a bit chubby,' they might say, pinching the imaginary inch (more like a millimetre) around their waists, 'I just hold off the chocolate for a couple of weeks and I'm back to normal.'

Well, bully for them! For many of us, it's a lot more complicated.

Airbrushing, food giants, hormones: is it my fault or isn't it?

This book isn't about the reasons behind the obesity 'epidemic' but I do want to put it in context - for me, the question of why so many of us have become overweight is an important one, and it's also relevant because it taps into the reasons I think this way of eating is working for many people when other 'diets' haven't.

The fact is, most of us in the West have access to all the right nutritious foods to keep our bodies healthy, without getting fat. But real lives are more complicated. I'll deal more with attitudes to food – and how this diet helps – in Chapter Four. But here's what Sally has to say about it:

I like the idea that no foods are sins. As a lifetime yo-yo dieter, I've found something that really works for me. It isn't too hard to fit it into my lifestyle as it's flexible, and if I

can't fast one day for any particular reason
(i.e. a social occasion) I don't feel that I've
failed. I just start again the next day.

Sally, 49

I'm the same: within a couple of weeks I no longer felt deprived, or guilty, or ruled by my appetite. Which meant weight loss became less about the psychology and more about the maths.

5:2: just a different way of eating less?

On the simplest level, 5:2 - or 6:1 or ADF – appears to work the same way as every other diet - you lose weight because you consume less energy (food) than you're using. The weight loss comes because, overall, you're eating less.

It doesn't sound very exciting - though some of the other physical and mental effects really are - but, ultimately, it's the same with all diets. It is possible that with fasting – as well as some other diets – there's what's known as a *metabolic advantage:* that is, eating this particular way will generate more weight loss (or, more specifically, *fat* loss) than can be attributed to the reduction in calories. But further research is needed.

Until we have more data, calories count on all diets. Take low-carbing. There's lots of talk about ketosis, which is a state where the body begins to access fat molecules for energy because it's deprived of the easier-to-process sugars it has access to when we eat carbohydrates. Those behind various low-carb regimes say that ketosis is one of the key factors in the weight losses observed by followers: it is seen by some almost as a 'magic' state.

However, many studies have shown that it's much more straightforward than that. Low-carb dieters are consuming fewer calories than they did before, simply because they've cut an entire food group out of their diet.

That's what happened to me when I did it. I ate less, without really thinking about it, because I had fewer choices. Yes, I could eat butter, which I love, but what was the point without crusty bread or a lovely hot baked potato? I didn't feel hungry, particularly, because protein tends to make you feel fuller, which is one advantage of a high-protein diet (there are potential disadvantages, too, as we'll see elsewhere). Of course, low-carb diets are also often high in fat, which is another factor: all that fat made me feel a bit sick after a while and I didn't want to eat anything at all. Therefore, I was eating less calories, almost by default.

But as soon as I started reintroducing the breads and potatoes into my diet (we moved to Spain, where bread is religion and potato-packed tortilla is the default vegetarian option), I was no more able to resist them than I was before.

I boomeranged right back to my previous weight. And then some.

The more extreme diets - Cabbage Soup, Maple Syrup, Grapefruit - cut your calorie intake by restricting your diet, but also your social life. Would anybody want to live on grapefruits for the rest of their life? I think it would feel like a very, very long life.

And as for cabbage soup...

The basic dieting equation:

**X (the energy your body needs to function) minus
Y (3,500 calories) =
Z (a weight loss of 1lb or 0.45kg)**

Hmm. As you can tell, algebra has never been my strong point. But simple arithmetic I *can* do.

And it works like this. It's estimated that to lose a pound of weight, we need to have a 'deficit' of 3,500 calories – the same figure applies to putting weight *on*. If we eat 3,500 more calories than we need – over any period of time – we will potentially weigh a pound (0.45 kg) more. That helps to explain why even eating one more biscuit a day, for example, can lead to significant weight gain over a year. On the positive side, means small changes to reduce our daily consumption – cutting out sugar in hot drinks, say – can have impressive cumulative effects.

So, to become a pound (0.45 kg) lighter, you must eat 3,500 less calories than your body needs (throughout this book, when I refer to calories, I'm referring to what nutrition labels list as kilo calories or kcal.). Eat 35,000 calories fewer and that's ten pounds (4.5 kg) gone.

That's the theory. As with everything in the diet/nutrition world, not everyone accepts it's quite that simple. John Briffa, who I mentioned before, believes that 'not all calories are equal' (bit.ly/TtdVta) in that protein calories keep your appetite sated for longer, and fat calories have their own advantages over 'carbohydrate calories' in terms of how they make you metabolise the fat stored in your body.

Another factor in how much weight we might lose is exercise – we're encouraged to exercise as part of a healthy living plan, but if you develop muscle, that mass will be denser and heavier than fat.

For the sake of our sums, however, let's keep it simple and work with the 3,500 as it gives us a baseline, and it's clear we do need to reduce what we're eating, i.e. create a deficit to burn our stored fat. The question is, how do you achieve this deficit?

For my entire dieting life, I've assumed that you must diet *all the time:* and that's where it's become tricky, because it's so hard to deny yourself all the foodie pleasures, and to stick to the regime when all you can see ahead is more deprivation.

All that time, there has been another way

5:2 – and all other types of intermittent fasting/ calorie restriction – offer a radically different, though obvious approach. If you reduce your calorie intake more drastically, but for a limited period, you'll lose the weight. It might be a little more gradual, but because you aren't denying yourself the pleasures of food the whole time, you stand a much higher chance of staying on track.

> *I've never really tried a formal diet before. I saw the 'Horizon' and decided it looked interesting. Had noticed my weight had been going up - tight clothes, roll of belly when I tied my shoes etc. Now I stick to an average of 600 calories, three days a week with no major problems.*
>
> *John, 58*

> *I've found it a relatively painless way of losing weight compared to others. To my mind the big benefit is the 5:2 is far easier*

to fit round family life/socialising etc. as one doesn't have to worry about it for the vast proportion of the time. My other half is a chef, and having smaller portions or calorie counting 7 days a week just ain't going to happen, but I can manage 2.

Sarah, 49

Doing the math(s)

A moderately active, average-sized woman needs 1800-2000 calories per day to maintain her weight, while for men it's 2300-2500 (I give instructions for calculating your exact needs later in Step One of Part Two).

Let's use Miss or Mrs Average as an example for now.

2000 (daily requirement) x 7 (days of the week) = 14,000 (total calorie needs to maintain weight)

So, if you're overweight and want to lose a pound a week (which many doctors suggest as a 'sustainable' weight loss – and which will also avoid you looking drawn, which can happen if you rush weight loss), you'd have to lower your intake by 3,500 calories i.e. consume a maximum of **10,500 in one week – which is 1,500 calories per day.**

Conventional calorie restricted diet:

7 days at 1,500 calories per day

Weekly Total = 10,500 calories

That's actually a higher allowance than many calorie-controlled diets, but it still represents a big drop from what you may be used to. It also means calorie counting every day for a very long period: with a stone (14 lbs or 6.4 kg) to lose, for example, you're talking about fourteen weeks of counting and deprivation. If you're looking to lose four stone (25 kg), you're potentially facing over a year of constantly obsessing over what you're eating.

Here's how it works on 5:2: you cut the calories more drastically, but only two days of the week. The rest of the time you eat normally.

5 x Feast Days of eating normally (approx. 2000 calories) =
10,000 calories
2 x Fast Days at 500 calories (25% of daily energy need) =
1000 calories
Weekly total: 11,000

OK, so the more mathematically aware reader will have spotted that under this example, you're eating 500 cals more than you would by calorie counting every day. This would potentially slow down weight loss slightly, though many dieters I've spoken to say that on Feast Days, they tend to naturally eat a little less – so I suspect it evens out.

> *I can fast because I know next day I can have chocolate AND wine if I so wish. Funnily enough, because I can, I don't binge.*
>
> *Myfanwy, 49*

The crucial thing about 5:2 is that for many dieters, it's so much easier to stick to those two days of being very careful, interspersed with five of relaxing and not being 'on a diet' at all. For those of us who have had success, that's what is keeping us going.

And, of course, if you decide to do the diet more often than two days a week – every other day, for example, (known as Alternate Daily Fasting or ADF) – the calorie deficit increases. So fasting on Sunday, Tuesday and Thursday looks like this:

4 x Feast Days- approx. 2000 calories – 8,000 calories

3 x Fast Days (25% of daily energy needs) = 1500
<u>Weekly Total: 9,500 calories</u>

On ADF the next week the situation could be reversed:
4 x Fast Days = 2,000
3 x Feast Days = 6,000
<u>Weekly Total: 8,000 calories</u>

Many people on ADF do stick to three Fast Days – but it's advisable that you don't fast more often than every other day, to avoid making more extreme metabolic changes that could end up working against you as you try to lose weight and improve your health. But if you stick to the guidelines outlined in the book, that won't be a problem.

What are the Fast Days like?

I won't lie – they can take some getting used to at first. We're so used to eating before we get anywhere near experiencing hunger that it can be odd or even alarming to begin with when our appetite kicks in.

I can't say I particularly look forward to

Fast Days, but they aren't too hard and I have always kept to them so far. I have blood-sugar issues, so have to ensure I do eat something in the morning, although I would rather not eat until lunch time or later.

Steph, 49

It's easy, and the more you do it, the easier it gets. Eat some protein on your restricted days, give the regime at least a month before considering if it works for you or not.

Paul, 47

500 calories for women – and 600 for men – is enough to keep you from feeling unwell, especially if you choose your foods wisely: much more on this, including easy recipes and ready-made meal suggestions, in Part Three.

Plus, believe it or not, hunger isn't a huge deal. When was the last time you felt hungry, instead of thirsty or bored? Allowing yourself to experience hunger - and then to satisfy it again - could be one of the most useful experiences when it comes to learning how to control your appetite and your eating.

Finally, and crucially, *it's only one day at a time.* In contrast to the daily monotony of 'normal' diets, with 5:2 you're only having to limit yourself for a couple of days (and they're not consecutive). I promise you, it's so much easier to say no to a cake or a glass of wine when you know you can have it tomorrow than it is when your diet feels like a very long punishment for being fat.

Weight loss is only the start...

So, that's the basic maths behind the diet. It involves a shift in how you think about dieting, and it's one that has the potential to make big changes. Various studies (1.usa.gov/fLnc4v) have shown that intermittent calorie restriction can be every bit as effective as conventional 'everyday' dieting – and that it can be easier to stick to!

On the weight loss front, there's also some suggestion that fasting may change how the body responds to the deficit, so you burn more fat that on other diets. Insulin – which is produced when you eat carbohydrates to release the sugar as energy – inhibits the body from using the stored body fat as energy. The less insulin in your system, the more you can use more of your own fat as 'fuel' to see you through the day. There's a good overview via this link (again, don't forget all the links are on my website for ease of access or type in this link bit.ly/V53n52).

The Big Question

Do 5:2 diets – or other forms of fasting – have effects *beyond* cutting calories and weight loss? There is growing evidence that they do. Increasingly, research suggests that limiting your eating dramatically for short periods may do some incredible things to your body, such as encourage it to heal itself, minimise the damage caused by our lifestyles and even protect or boost growth in our brain cells.

How? As we'll see in the "science bit" in Chapter Three, the secret's in your cells and your genes.

But before we get to the Science Bit, here's how I got on in the first week of my 5:2 experiment...

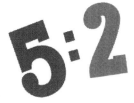

First Fast – of many?

Mood: excited, apprehensive, unsure

I'm taking the plunge. Fasting is the future… maybe.

My boyfriend is sceptical, and other friends (who haven't seen the programme) are also dubious - one talked in dark tones about 'starvation mode' where your body responds to cutting calories by slowing down all its systems to keep you alive: they say when you go back to eating normal amounts, you put even more weight on.

But from the little research I've managed to do online, it looks like the 'intermittent' part of intermittent calorie restriction will stop the dreaded starvation mode, because you're never fasting for long enough to send your body into a panic.

If in doubt, *Google* it...

As I am self-employed, and work from home, my first response to pretty much all my daily decisions is to Google them. Seriously. It's not something I'm proud of - recently I've asked the big G where to rent a holiday cottage, how to answer my brand new but complicated mobile phone, and whether it's true that Marilyn Monroe was severely flatulent (apparently so). So it's inevitable that it'd be the same with my latest diet project.

The TV show was fascinating, but I still have lots of questions: how many meals a day should I eat on the 'fast' days - is it better to eat one or three? What should my calorie target be on those days? Can I *really* eat as much as I like on my unrestricted or 'feed days'?

I fully expected to find lots of sites dealing with this approach, but what's out there seems really unfocused - either scientific papers or some very hyped-sounding e-books, costing lots and lots of dollars.

There does seem to be plenty of information to back up the potential health benefits, though - so I'm giving it a whirl.

It All Adds Up

The first thing I have to do is work out roughly how many calories I need to maintain my current (over)weight - I do this via the MyFitnessPal website, which I already have as an app on my phone. It's a very neat site which, so far, has mainly helped me track how much I'm eating - too much - and given me reasons to feel guilty about my lack of self-control. *How* many glasses of cava?

My first step is to work out my Basal Metabolic Rate - that's an estimate of how many calories someone of my size, height and age might need just to get through the day. There are at least two different formulas as well, and disagreement about which is more accurate. I plump for one formula and get 1,365 which is a terrifyingly low figure...

Until I realise it's the absolute baseline and I have to now use that figure multiplied by a factor depending on how active I am. This latest sum is called the Harris Benedict Formula - which sounds a bit like an episode of Sherlock - but involves multiplying my BMR by a number relating to my activity levels.

Little/no exercise:
    BMR * 1.2 = Total Calorie Need
Light exercise:
    BMR * 1.375 = Total Calorie Need
Moderate exercise (3-5 days/wk):
    BMR * 1.55 = Total Calorie Need
Very active (6-7 days/wk):
    BMR * 1.725 = Total Calorie Need
Extra active (very active & physical job):
    BMR * 1.9 = Total Calorie Need

I'm going for light exercise and decide, to be safe, to pick the lowest figure.

So 1365 x 1.375 = 1876.875

That, it seems, is the amount I should be eating every day to maintain my current weight. Most low-cal diets I've followed start at about 1,000 cals a day so 1877 sounds pretty generous.

Goodness knows what I've been eating per day to put this much weight on…

The third calculation is the killer though – for this new regime to actually count as a fast (and potentially bring me all the health benefits that scientists are researching) I have to divide my calorie needs by 25%.

Which is a slightly scary 469.25 – even lower than the averages of 500 for women and 600 for men that presenter Dr Michael Mosley quoted on his programme. (There's a full guide to doing this yourself in Step One of Part Two) I go to the fridge and start reading labels – on ready meals, soups, fruit and veg packaging.

Yes, it's low. But it's also… possibly … doable.

Little and How Often?

The final decision is about how often I'm going to calorie restrict. I've read Michael Mosley's tweets. Originally he did 5:2 - so five days eating normally, two of very limited calories, on Tuesday and Thursday. But his weight loss has been so successful that he's down to 6:1. Other people online are trying alternate days, so fast-feast-fast, but I'm a bit daunted by that. Although of course Alternate Day Fasting is self-limiting, in that you'll still eat properly every other day - I don't know how I'll cope with even a single day of eating less than 500 calories in total.

5:2 sounds good to begin with. Now all I need to do is, well, start…

Fast Day 1: August 9 2012

I wake up and try to pretend it's a normal day. A normal day where I happen to limit myself to a quarter of what my body needs, energy wise, and probably about a sixth of what I usually give it!

For breakfast I eat what I usually eat – a fruit and yogurt combo I got to like when I low-carbed, and one that usually keeps me from feeling hungry till lunchtime. Trouble is, my usual portion size would take up more than half my calorie requirement for the day. So with the help of my digital scales, I measure out a doll-sized breakfast. If you've never tried measuring out 25g of yogurt, it's approximately one fifth of a small pot. Not very much. I use a tiny bowl and savour all four tea-spoonfuls.

I've bought a big bottle of sparkling water, as my main 'treat'– also, I know as a diet veteran that staying hydrated is super-important. Looks like these are the only bubbles I'll be getting today…

As lunchtime approaches, my mood is not best helped by a rejection letter from the Women's Institute where I'd auditioned to be one of the speakers on their official list. I'd given talks to them in the past, but at my audition, the 100-strong panel decided I wasn't up to it – though they do say I had a clear speaking voice and a pleasant personality.

Hmm. Good job they can't see my grumpy face now, as I stand in the kitchen with the letter in one hand, the other one hovering over the packet of HobNobs.

But no.

I am better than that! And *pleasant,* too.

I make myself a calorie-free black coffee and try not to think about lunch.

The Department of Weights and Measures

Weighing is good displacement activity. That, and reading the labels on the back of ready meals. There is, frankly, not much fun in cooking with so few calories to play with, but I did spot a Butternut Squash dish in Marks & Spencer with just 140 calories for half a pack. OK, I think it's meant as a side dish, but it's quite filling for lunch and also allows me to treat myself to five cherry tomatoes, some rocket leaves and a teaspoon full of balsamic vinegar as a dressing.

And, to keep it simpler, I have the same for dinner. Why mess with a winning formula? Dessert is the same as breakfast. And the total: 463 calories! Three under, should have had a couple more rocket leaves…

Time for bed

How's it been? Well, I've got a slight headache and have felt more peckish than hungry. Portions are small but it's been easy because the man of the house is out with mates tonight, so I haven't had to cook or resist sharing some wine.

But mainly it's been easy because I know I can eat exactly what I want tomorrow. I go to bed early - my tummy is rumbling, but my conscience is clear, and I hope to dream of what I can eat for breakfast in just over 12 hours' time.

<u>What I ate to the last gram:</u>

Breakfast

Greek-Style Natural Yogurt, 25 g:34 cals

Ground Almonds 4g:25 cals

Strawberries - Raw, 53 g: 17 cals

<u>Lunch</u>

M & S Moroccan Butternut Wedges With Roast
Vegetables, 1/2 pack:140 cals

Peppery Baby leaf Rocket Salad, 20 g: 4
cals

Balsamic Vinegar of Modena, 5 ml: 5 cals

Cherry Tomatoes, 5 tomatoes:15 cals

<u>Dinner</u>

M & S Moroccan Butternut Wedges With Roast
Vegetables, 1/2 pack:140 cals

Cherry Tomatoes, 5 tomatoes:12 cals

Generic - Balsamic Vinegar, 0.25 tbs:3 cals

<u>Snacks</u>

Greek-Style Natural Yogurt, 19 g:25 cals

Ground Almonds, 5 g:31 cals

Strawberries - Raw, 63 g Calories: 12cals

Total for day: 463 cals

Chapter Three: The Fasting Recharge - make y body work better, and last longer

As we established in Chapter Two, slimmer people tend to live longer. So if you're carrying too much weight, it makes sense to lose some.

But one of the major appeals for intermittent dieters, whether they're doing 5:2, 6:1 or alternate day fasting, is the potential for huge health benefits which scientists believe exceed those that weight reduction would offer on its own.

> *I have concerns over dementia as it runs in my family so this side was particularly appealing. I also liked the idea that the diet was "part time" as I enjoy food and it is an important part of my family/social life as well as a hobby.*
>
> *Kirsty, 38*

> *Started fasting in earnest and have lost a stone in six weeks. Not strictly ADF, but tend to do 3/7 rather than 2/7. This works because:- 1. I like the science behind it and 2. I tell myself I can eat tomorrow.*
>
> *Linda, 52*

bers of studies on both humans *and*
that there are unique benefits to be gained
from fasting or restricting your calorie intake quite
severely, *even if you only do it some of the time.*

Common sense might suggest that depriving the
body of nutrients would be damaging and, indeed, it does
put the body under stress.

But it's the body's response to that stress that seems
to hold the key to the health benefits – just as a stressful
job can bring out the best in us and help us achieve more,
putting your body under stress in a controlled way, can
encourage it to heal itself and trigger processes that protect
and repair.

Time for the "science bit": the secret is in the cells...

The science bit is short, and sweet, and if you want to
understand why this diet might have such huge benefits,
it's worth focusing on this part! But do feel free to skip this
part – or any part – of the book if you're not in the mood
for theory. Part Two is the practical part, and I want you to
use, and abuse, the guide as it suits you. No rules,
remember?

Still with me? OK. We're all made up of cells –
approximately 100 million *million* of them in total. Think
of TV images of 'test tube babies' and IVF where you can
see the cells doubling in number over and over again, as
the embryo develops.

Our cells continue their hard work throughout our
lives. There are approximately two hundred different
kinds, all with different functions – and they're being
replaced at the rate of millions per second. Some cells are
constantly replaced, though others can't be. Even those
that do multiply can only do so a certain number of times.
It's this ceiling that is responsible for ageing – as the
number of skin cells drops, for example, your skin becomes
thinner.

As part of their life cycle, some cells will also self-
destruct, in a carefully controlled house-keeping process
known as apoptosis (read more at: bit.ly/4oz2RD) – they'll
even 'tidy up' after themselves so they don't leave behind
anything that could damage other cells. I love the idea of
them being all Girl Guide-ish to the last minute...

Another important process is autophagy
(bit.ly/Ya4EgO) – literally 'self-eating': this process can
lead to the death of a cell but may also help it to survive
under stress.

But sometimes the cell production and destruction
process goes wrong: when too many are produced,

uncontrollably, it causes tumours. The kind that then invade neighbouring tissues are malignant – in other words, cancerous.

Meanwhile, damage to brain cells can cause Alzheimer's or other forms of dementia, as the structure of brain cells is changed: they may die or become tangled up, and the chemical messengers that pass information around the brain no longer work as hard.

Living Causes Ageing

The trouble with life is that the very process of living causes damage to the body.

Cells are damaged by the processes involved in producing the energy we need to function – our bodies break down food into glucose (the simplest form of sugar) to use as energy, but that breaking down also damages proteins in the body and causes many of the signs and symptoms of old age.

Oxygen is part of that process but while the body makes the energy, it's also producing free radicals which attack your cells in a process known as oxidative stress. When we're younger, we can cope better with this, 'mopping up' the free radicals before they do too much damage. But it catches up with us sooner or later...

Can eating less slow this down?

So, if you produce less energy, then maybe you're also causing less damage. That's one of the fundamental issues at the heart of much anti-ageing research.

It's been demonstrated in animal studies – from fruit flies to worms, mice to dogs – that eating less, or less frequently, can prolong their lives.

The exact chemical and biological processes involved are being researched, but the studies have already led to many people choosing to eat less than their calorie requirements, all the time – not just to keep their weight down, but to increase their lifespans.

As someone with a keen interest in diets and nutrition, I've read a lot about Calorie Restrictors – these people typically eat only 70-80% of their recommended intake, though they take extra care to eat very nutritious foods. Many people end up with BMIs 19, 18 or lower, and frequently show reduced blood pressure and cholesterol levels. One of the main movements is called Calorie Restriction with Optimum Nutrition – which is why they're known as CRONIES.

However, what I had read and viewed on TV about CRONIES had put me off - the guy featured in the fasting programme seems fairly typical in that his diet looked expensive and pretty wasteful - he kept the skin of fruit for example but discarded the pulp. And though he was very healthy, living that way all the time didn't look much fun!

Now it seems 5:2 and Alternate Day Calorie Restriction may offer the benefits of that CRONIE lifestyle – but in a much more civilised and laid back form. Instead of having to watch calories obsessively all the time, we can do it in short, sharp bursts that encourage the body to activate all the protective and reparative processes that may help us live longer and better.

It's not just how much you eat, it's also what you eat

Different food stuffs also have different effects on the body – we've already mentioned that producing glucose stimulates those damaging free radicals.

According to the 'Horizon' show, protein in particular seems to turbo-charge the cell production process. The scientist interviewed, Professor Valter Longo, compared our bodies to racing cars where protein is making the cars race faster - what Dr Mosley called Go-Go Mode - with no chance at all to retune or recharge. Driving at high speed the whole time without ever putting the cars in for service causes wear and tear – and so if we eat constantly, we're effectively increasing the wear and tear on our bodies.

So what fasting or severely limiting calories appears to do is put our bodies in for a service. We deprive our body of calories - fuel - and that way, instead of making the body produce new cells, we encourage it to take stock - and take care of - the cells it already has.

IGF-1 – the 1 to watch?

IGF-1 is a growth hormone that many scientists in this field believe is central to the effects of this diet, *and* to both the ageing process and the development of cancers. IGF-1 stands for Insulin-Like Growth Factor and it plays an important role in children's growth. But once we're adults, the effects may not be so positive: in particular, the hormone seems to lock us into this constant cycle of regrowth that may not do us any favours, the *go-go* mode Dr Mosley talked about.

There's firm evidence in animal studies that lower levels of IGF-1 can lead to better health and longer life expectancy: mice on a diet of either continuous calorie restriction or intermittent calorie restriction have been shown to live 40% longer than mice fed a normal diet (bit.ly/Sh2rtO): that would be the equivalent of a person living to 120 or more!

Indeed, a recent report also suggests that a hormone that blocks the action of IGF-1 might in future offer some of the longevity benefits of fasting or calorie restriction – without having to fast! A group of mice were genetically engineered to produce constant supplies of a hormone usually produced during fasting, FGF21. The experiment extended their lifespan by a third (bit.ly/RNNDnI) although fertility and bone density where affected.

Of course, we need to be wary of assuming that what works in mice will work for us. One clue comes from a rare *human* genetic condition known as Laron syndrome, where very low levels of IGF-1 are produced. People with the mutation don't grow very tall, but the lack of the hormone also has very strong protective effects against cancer and diabetes. Professor Longo from the University of Southern California – the same guy who gave us the car analogy above - monitored 99 people with the condition in Ecuador with astonishing results.

To date, they've now been followed for twenty-four years, and none of them have developed diabetes, and only one has been diagnosed with non-fatal cancer. Yet 5% of their neighbours – with similar diets and lifestyles - have been diagnosed with diabetes, and 17% had cancer diagnosed during that same period. Overall, the Laron syndrome group didn't live longer, but that may be down to the high number of accidents caused by being smaller.

One pointer towards the possible protective effects of low-levels of IGF-1 came when the scientists studied blood serum from those with the Laron mutation under the microscope. Cells suffered less DNA damage than 'normal' blood cells from non Laron patients when they were exposed to a toxin. Yet when the scientists added IGF-1 – that protection disappeared.

Food and IGF-1

So if IGF-1 is a contributor to DNA damage – the kind we talked about when we were discussing Free Radicals and Oxidative stress - then what happens when we eat less and consequently produce less IGF-1?

It seems that as levels of the hormone drop, the body goes into the repair mode we mentioned before.

The SIRT1 Gene – Gene Genius of anti-ageing?

One of the key genes anti-ageing scientists are focusing on is the SIRT1 gene, which produces a protein called Sirtuin (silent mating type information regulation 2 homolog: don't worry, there won't be a test at the end).

It certainly works for yeast and worms. Having extra copies of this gene extends their lifespans.

In human-focused research, there's been attention paid to the effect of calorie restriction in activating the gene, and all the 'repair mode' benefits we've been discussing in this chapter.

The theory goes that Sirtuin may play a part in regulating/improving the processes we've discussed above, including apoptosis (regulated cell death), reducing damage by 'free radicals' and also reducing what's known as inflammatory response. That's where the body tries to protect itself from infection – it works well when you have a cut or a minor infection, and various infection-fighting cells cause inflammation including redness and swelling as they race to the location to fight the infection. But it's not good news when your body overall stays in this inflamed state – in fact, it's thought chronic inflammation might be responsible for many medical conditions, including cancers, heart disease and arthritis.

SIRT1 may be responsible for many of the benefits seen in animals and humans – and it can be activated by calorie restriction, including 5:2 and ADF diets. Further research is ongoing into this – and into the possibility that you can also give your SIRT1 gene a boot up the backside with... red wine?

The Wine Connection

The skin and pips of grapes contain a molecule called resveratrol – and some scientists believe this might partly explain the 'French Paradox' – where studies have shown some French citizens live longer than other Western Europeans, despite diets high in fat.

But before you crack open the Merlot, the research is ongoing – billions of dollars are being spent trying to use this knowledge to develop life-extending treatments. Yet the role of the resveratrol – and the SIRT1 gene in general - in increasing lifespans is still controversial.

Plastic surgeon, James Johnson, whose UpDayDownDay Diet can be seen as a stricter, more regulated version of the flexible approaches to Alternate Day Fasting described in this book, suggests that resveratrol supplements (which he sells via his website) can activate the gene alongside calorie restriction.

His book is interesting, and goes into far more detail about the science than this book. However, on a personal level, I don't believe I would have begun this diet had I only read his version – he advocates the use of diet shakes to kick-start the activation of SIRT1 and the weight loss, whereas for many of us, that's not an appealing prospect – I'll talk more about making food choices to maximise your chances of success in Part Three.

Uncertainties and further research

The precise mechanisms of SIRT1, resveratrol and IGF-1 in the fasting process are still unclear, but there are numerous studies showing the potential beneficial effects of ADF and calorie restriction on different medical conditions.

Some research is incomplete and ongoing – but for me (and for many of the scientists involved), there's enough evidence from different sources to suggest this is worth pursuing, which reinforces my personal view that weight loss is only part of the appeal of the 5:2 life.

Research Overview

Much of the evidence at this stage either comes from animal studies, because human lifespans are so much longer and therefore the studies take longer too. So where humans have tried ADF or Calorie Restricted Diets, the effects are often measured by the results of blood tests that indicate the likelihood of developing certain diseases, e.g. insulin sensitivity for diabetes, LDL and HDL cholesterol for heart disease, peak flow testing for asthma.

The best overview I've found is by Krista Varady – who featured in the 'Horizon' programme – and Marc Hellerstein. Their review of studies was published in 2007 so is a little out of date, but contains a great summary of the diverse research: (bit.ly/X4rXHs). Krista was featured talking about the ADF version she tested – and you can find online interviews with her at bit.ly/9nru75

There's a more recent review available via bit.ly/qyQri2 also explores health benefits – and disadvantages – of the kinds of fasts advocated for religious reasons.

Cancer

In animal trials, there are signs that ADF (and Calorie Restriction) has inhibited the growth of certain cancer cells, and improved response to anti-cancer therapy.

Meanwhile the Genesis Breast Cancer Prevention Centre (genesisuk.org) in Manchester has been measuring the effects of an intermittent calorie restriction diet, similar to the 5:2 diet, in women with a high risk of developing the disease.

Because excess weight is often associated with an increased risk of breast cancer, lowering weight can reduce the risk by up to 40%. Even more crucially, this form of dieting might offer extra benefits at genetic level. Their first study was encouraging and highlighted that the intermittent restriction appeared to be at least as effective as continuous (everyday) dieting in weight loss terms

(1.usa.gov/113kSH6). Those on intermittent diets also showed greater 'insulin sensitivity' than the everyday dieters – which is a good thing in terms of diabetes prevention.

The BRRIDE (Breast Risk Reduction Intermittent Diet Evaluation) study has been completed even more recently and has analysed breast and body tissues to see if the diet has made changes to how the genes are behaving. The hope is that that a diet of 1,800 calories five days a week, and 600 calories two days a week, may reduce the activity of the SCD gene which is thought to be a factor in the development of breast cancer.

As I said in the introduction, a very high percentage of the female relatives on my mother's side of the family have had breast cancer diagnoses. Apart from my regular mammograms, I've felt powerless in the face of this history. Until now – the evidence may not yet be there in black and white but I am doing this diet with an eye on future research and I await the outcome of this study with particularly keen interest. You can download a summary of this important work via bit.ly/U4DbEH

Heart Disease

In animal studies, rodents saw a decrease in blood pressure, heart rate and cardiovascular disease risk indicators when they were put on ADF regimes. In another experiment on rats, the damage caused when a heart attack was induced was less in those on ADF.

In a human study, there was shown to be no effect on blood pressure, but Krista Varady's studies of people who did ADF (with one 500 or 600 calorie meal on Fasting days) showed levels of LDL (or 'bad') cholesterol in their blood fell, as did blood pressure in some cases. And it's something also reported by some of our 5:2 dieters:

> *Lost half a stone, BP down to the point where I can reduce my BP medication. Cholesterol has come down from 6.1 to 5.2.*
>
> *Paul, 47*

> *I was initially drawn to watching the 'Horizon' programme because of the weight loss but after watching, the weight loss just seemed to be a fortunate side effect. Now my blood pressure has lowered slightly.*
>
> *Claire, 43*

Asthma, auto- immune disorders and other chronic conditions

Dr James Johnson, whose book I mentioned earlier, has carried out research on people with asthma undertaking his version of the diet, and found that 19 out of 20 people who followed it saw improvements in their symptoms (bit.ly/Uuec1Z).

His studies of over 500 people who've followed his Alternate Day regime has also shown self-reported improvements in a range of medical conditions including "insulin resistance, asthma, seasonal allergies, infectious diseases of viral, bacterial and fungal origin, autoimmune disorder (rheumatoid arthritis), osteoarthritis, symptoms due to CNS inflammatory lesions (Tourette's, Meniere's) cardiac arrhythmias (PVCs, atrial fibrillation), menopause-related hot flashes."

That'll be flushes, to us in the UK. Certainly, a number of the people I know who are doing 5:2 have noticed improvements, even to long-standing health issues.

> *Weight is coming off, I look better in clothes and the rheumatoid arthritis in my hands doesn't hurt so much, and I have more movement in my fingers without them cracking. Will be interested to see how the blood pressure is when I see the doctor next.*
> *Anita, 51*

I had some quite severe menopausal problems and whilst I did not particularly expect the diet to make any difference, it was a nice surprise to find that it does. My night sweats have stopped and whilst I get the occasional hot flush, they're not nearly as bad as they were.

Sally, 49

Anecdotal evidence, of course, but interesting, too.

Diabetes

I've seen first-hand how Type 2 (or 'late onset') diabetes is not the minor inconvenience many people assume it to be. In many cases, this kind of diabetes strikes in middle-age, though increasing obesity levels mean it's affecting people at earlier and earlier ages. The condition can cause sight problems, kidney disease, circulation issues, nerve problems and sometimes it even necessitates amputation of the lower limbs.

There's also more awareness now of changes that occur in the lead up to developing diabetes, as the body becomes less sensitive to the insulin that regulates sugar in the blood. *Insulin sensitivity* is a *good* thing as it means the body responds well to the insulin the pancreas is producing.

For many years, dieting wisdom has favoured 'grazing' as a way of eating, so that you snack between meals and never allow yourself to get hungry. But that also means that your body is constantly having to produce insulin to regulate sugar levels in the blood.

It makes sense to me, as a non-scientist, that reducing the number of sugar/insulin spikes you experience during the day may be better for the body. Insulin is also lipogenic – which means that while it's in circulation, your body lays down fat stores, instead of burning fat – another reason why dieters would want to reduce too many spikes.

Animal studies (particularly on rats) certainly suggest that ADF may have a positive effect on how we process glucose – but human trials are less clear, and there's a suggestion that men may benefit more than women. However, the Genesis cancer study outlined above found that women who followed an intermittent calorie restriction regime showed bigger improvements in their insulin sensitivity than those who followed a traditional diet: see this link, 1.usa.gov/113kSH6 for more.

It's hard to draw firm conclusions at this stage but on a personal level, I am encouraged by the potential to reduce the risk. Of course, losing weight by any means also reduces the risk of developing Type 2 Diabetes in overweight and obese people, which for me is enough of a benefit for now.

Gender differences

For many years, medical research tended to assume that female bodies worked the same as male ones – so they carried out research on men and applied the findings to both.

There's more recognition now that this can lead to false conclusions, and there are specific concerns around whether women – especially during their fertile years – may not respond in the same positive ways to ADF or intermittent calorie restriction. Sleep disturbance and a reduction in fertility have been noted in female subjects of research.

The more aware we are of the possible pros as well as cons of this diet, the better. Of course, it has to be a personal decision.

If you want to know more on this particular topic, there are two blog articles (go to bit.ly/Uueru8 and bit.ly/11jrlwF or follow the links from my downloadable links).

What about Starvation Mode?

Over the years, the idea of Starvation Mode has been a scary prospect for all dieters: as I said in my diary entry, friends mentioned it to me when I began this diet.

The concern is that if the body is deprived of food for a lengthy period, it will take emergency action, effectively 'rationing' the number of calories it uses and becoming so efficient in using them that if you then go back to eating normally, you will put more weight on, because your body is being over efficient.

In other words, starvation mode might have protected Stone Age Man (and woman!) from premature death – but it might also stop 21st century man and woman ever fitting into those skinny jeans...

It is very hard to work out what's fact and what's fiction when it comes to this 'mode' – some diet gurus refer to it as a myth, others hold it up as the bogeyman of dieters. The process of changing how the body fuels itself is also known as 'adaptive thermogenesis' – i.e. your body adapts to the reduced calories by changing how energy is produced. Ultimately, a human body deprived of food for a long time – 72 hours or more, though opinions vary – will begin to break down cells to produce what it needs and that's likely to mean muscle mass will decrease, the longer the starvation lasts. That's *not* a good thing.

The key words here appear to be **lengthy period -** which is the beauty of the 5:2 approach. Not only does intermittent calorie restriction help with willpower - you only have to resist temptation till you're back OFF the diet tomorrow - it also prevents any real risk of entering into Starvation Mode because you're not restricting calories for long enough to (non-medical term here) freak your body out.

Which has to be good news for your bikini body - and your hard-working cells.

> *I needed to get my cholesterol down, as the doctor was concerned about it. I also wanted to look and feel better. It seems that you're not allowed to admit you're doing this for anything other than the health benefits, but actually I do want to feel better about how I look. I've been doing it just over a month and lost 15 pounds. I can now get into a smaller bra. I've also had to search out some smaller trousers.*
>
> *Sally 49*

> *I've lost seventeen pounds. A new dress I ordered arrived today and when I unwrapped it, I thought, 'I'll NEVER get*

into that!' It looks more like a 10 than the 12
I ordered. Anyway, it fits like a glove.
That's the thing I like about this 'diet': I
seem to have lost the weight in exactly the
places I wanted to lose – stomach, bum and
hips.

Janie, 49

Mind and Body...

So overall, the potential benefits of fasting for your physical health could be significant. But is that going to be enough to boost your willpower when you're craving chocolate at 4pm?

In Chapter Four, I'll look at how fasting re-educates your appetite and your mental attitude, and how it also appears to have beneficial effects on brain cells, potentially reducing your risk of Alzheimer's disease and other forms of dementia.

Before we delve into this, I've got one fast under my belt – now what about the rest of my life? Read on for the next instalment of my diet diary...

Kate's 5:2 Diary Part Three: August & September 2012

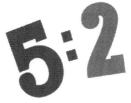

MyFitnessPal keeps shouting at me

Mood: excited, curious, lucky

So. One fast down, the rest of my life to go…

The day after my first Fast Day feels amazing - and I must admit I go a bit OTT on the food. The TV show says you can eat pretty much what you want on your non-diet days so… well, I behaved myself till tea-time - even cutting my yogurt breakfast right down - but then it all went a bit Thank God It's Friday Night Now Let's Eat Everything in the Fridge…

I started well, with a blueberry and yogurt breakfast at just 104 cals, then had a Panini at lunchtime. But at dinner…

Italian Rose Wine, 500 ml: 300 cals
Millionaire's Shortbread Dessert: 440 cals

Tortilla Chips, 25 g: 119 cals
Edamame, Pea and Wasabi Dip, 125 g: 208 cals
Wholemeal Roll: 155 cals
Garlic Mushrooms 100 g:135 cals
Cherry Tomatoes, 5 tomatoes 60g 12 cals
Country Life Butter 10 g 69 cals
Graze Box - Toffee Apple 68 cals

Total 1,910 cals

I'm a bit ashamed to post it all. There's a dessert here that almost totalled my entire calorie consumption yesterday plus almost two-thirds of a bottle of wine (I am celebrating *not* being on a Fast Day?).

And yet… I need to be honest: we all have our bad days and it still came to only a little bit more than the 1876 I'd worked out is what I could eat without gaining any more weight.

I'm definitely not going to monitor all of my feast days, but it's almost reassuring to know that on this diet I can eat all of those rather yummy things - now and then - and still potentially lose weight if I am careful on the Fast Days. Speaking of which…

Fast Day 2 is a Saturday and I eat exactly the same as I ate on the first Fast Day. Which I thought would be boring but is actually pretty liberating. After all, it's only really in diet books that we have something different for breakfast every day, isn't it? So what's wrong with sticking to a formula that you know will stop you feeling ravenous?

August is party month!

I knew when I decided to embark on the diet that August wasn't going to be easy - I had lots of parties and events to go to, and so reasoned that my diet was a) going to be hard to follow and b) probably more about stopping the rot than helping me lose any weight. In total, I fast on seven days this month – and my expectations are realistic.

The Schoolmarm in my computer

MyFitnessPal is quite cross with me, though. On Fast Day, it tells me off for eating too little - saying I might go into starvation mode… luckily, all I've read about the science says that one day's fasting at a time won't affect my metabolism.

The strangest thing is that I've begun to *like* my Fast Days… even look forward to them. I feel it's a day off from thinking about food, and also a bit of a 'rest' for my body, which seems to fit in with what the programme said – that your body repairs itself while it's not running fast on protein.

I've been experimenting with eating at different times. With so much diabetes in my family, I wonder whether part of the benefit of fasting might be that your body isn't having to produce insulin all the time – and so maybe trying to eat fewer meals a day might be a good thing.

Just as strange is how hunger feels. I'd forgotten. Often what I'd mistaken for hunger is actually thirst or even boredom.

But now that I let myself get hungry on my Fast Days, it's not nearly as scary or overwhelming an experience as I feared. I'm aware that I am so lucky that I can avoid food for one or two days a week without worrying whether the food will be there when I want it to be. Eating less feels like a check-in - a reminder of what the right amount is to eat, and how fortunate we are that there will be food when we're ready.

Weight on 31 August: 156lbs - total lost so far, 5lbs
Days on diet: 22

Hooray! That's a bigger loss than I was expecting. My clothes are looser, my confidence that I can lose weight this way is increasing… Could this be what I've been looking for at last?

Souped-up September

Party month over, now it's back to reality. I like autumn and I like the chance to give the diet a proper go now. The five pounds (2.3kg) I lost last month is a great start and it also feels sustainable.

I'm now settling into a routine: Fast Days are Mondays and Wednesdays, so my weekends are free for eating out and enjoying myself without calorie counting.

I'm also skipping breakfast on my Fast Days, except for black coffee. And although I am a keen cook, on Fast Days I rely on very simple foods: salads, ready-made soups, perhaps some berries or yogurt. But it also means I can plan to enjoy doing some baking at the weekends, something that was completely out of bounds when I low-carbed or calorie-counted the whole time.

Not that the current calorie counting is a huge burden - am using MyFitnessPal but I'm getting to know by instinct what the right level of food is.

Beetroot Power

The weather changes mid-month, and I worry about switching from salads, to relying on soup. So I experiment with the chunkier ones you buy in pots in the supermarket. Even the ones with cheese or cream rarely contain more than 150 cals a portion, so they'll usually form the basis of my food for the day. I rather like that most of my food is contained in one pot: a Fast looks less daunting then somehow.

One of my choices is beetroot soup - I am surprised I haven't turned beetroot pink as my Fast Days often include some of the red peril - especially the 'sweet fire' spicy beetroot I can eat by the bucket load. Still, whatever works for me, eh?

On top of my daily soup ration, there's then room for a couple of 100 calorie snacks or treats: beetroot (!), some frozen berries with yogurt and a tiny amount of muesli for texture, a couple of apples, a banana, the world's smallest portion of tortilla chips. One evening I am meeting friends and don't want to cancel so I even allow myself a 100 calorie glass of wine. It does seem a bit decadent to be 'using' a fifth of my calories on alcohol but at least I'm a cheap date.

The doll's house portions are slightly surreal and maybe a bit sad - but because it's only a couple of days a week, I don't care too much. I can see how the measuring and weighing could become an obsession, and a not altogether healthy one, which is why

I think the days when you eat what you like are important for psychological, as well as physiological, reasons. It's about enjoying the pleasure of food, which is so often absent in a diet.

Feasting not feeding!

I've decided to call my 'eating' days 'Feast Days' - on the TV show, they called them 'feed' days which had a slightly farmyard feel about it, and also reminded me a bit of an article I'd read about 'feeders' - men who like to date larger women and watch as they eat a lot. Those two ideas aren't really fitting in with my hopes for this lifestyle, whereas 'feast' feels far better. The point is not to indulge in a Nigella-frenzy of cakes and puddings, but to savour the food on the days when you're free to eat what you like.

I also find that the early tendency to overdo it slightly on my 'feast' days is reducing as I get used to the diet. One reason is that after counting the calories the day before, I am more aware of what everything contains - so a chocolate brownie from Costa is something I choose to savour after a small lunch, rather than something I bolt down unnoticed as I run for the train. And it tasted so good…

The other reason is that all your senses are heightened after a day of fasting. Even a single slice of peanut butter on toast feels like a feast after a day on 500 calories…

Weight on 30 September: 152lbs
Total lost: 9lbs Days on Diet: 52

I slowed down a little so it's still not a dramatic weight loss, but at this rate, I should have lost a stone or more by Christmas, and be back into the healthy BMI zone.

It might not seem a huge breakthrough, but it really is. When I remember how I felt in July - that my weight and my attitude to food were out of control, that I had no way of 'stopping the rot' - I feel very lucky.

And, of course, I'm seeing the difference. My clothes are looser and even

my bra needs adjusting. Could the dreaded
back fat - one of those *Daily Mail*
obsessions - be facing its nemesis?

Roll on October...

Chapter Four: The Hunger Game - Fasting is Good for the Brain

Dieting is all in the mind...

Or at least, people who are successful in losing weight are those who have the mental strength to ignore cravings for long-term physical benefit. It's something I know many dieters - including myself - find difficult. If the body showed the results of that slice of chocolate cake overnight, it might be easier.

Our bodies are built to consume and conserve energy for survival. Pretty vital for early man, but in the industrialised 21st century, when many of us are lucky enough to have a vast choice and availability of food, making the 'right' choices about what we consume can be easier said than done. In theory, we have lots of appetising fresh produce available, and can make the right decisions: in practice, I know many of us feel out of control.

If you read the diary entries I've included in this ebook, you'll get a sense that my own weight issues result from a whole cocktail of factors:

o   switching from an active job to a sedentary one;

o   hating most forms of exercise;

o   a sweet tooth - and a savoury one, too;

o   a love of cooking, especially baking;

o   a slightly addictive personality;

o   a naturally, um, curvy body shape;

o   a strong association between food and reward. Which means that whenever I'm feeling a bit rubbish about how tight my jeans are, my first instinct is to head straight for the biscuit tin.

What's your reason?

How about you? Why not take a couple of minutes to think about the reasons you might not be making the right choices?

Do any of these ring a bell?

o   Stress - we lead busy lives, commute long distances, and work long hours: often we turn to food, particularly dishes high in fat or sugar, to provide fast energy boosts to meet a deadline or comfort ourselves after a hard day.

o   Commercial interests - manufacturers and retailers know that processed foods often generate higher profits, so these are marketed in ways that promote those energy boosting or comforting qualities: it's often easier to buy 'treat' foods or fast food when we're on the move than to try to buy or prepare fresher or unprocessed foods.

- o Mixed messages about what foods are healthy - with some foods labelled 'low fat' turning out to be high sugar, or vice versa.
- o Media images of beauty - including air-brushed photographs - present such perfect human specimens that we lose sight of what normal or healthy is - and when we can't live up to the impossible, we comfort ourselves with food.
- o Upbringing - our own attitudes to food as a reward or punishment will be closely related to our upbringing and those around us - offering biscuits or alcohol to 'compensate' for doing something unpleasant, or experiencing conflict, for example.
- o Hunger Phobia - we are often so busy 'grazing' or eating food throughout the day that we become terrified of feeling hungry even though for most of us in industrialised nations, it will only be a temporary state. Yet that constant feeding can also remove the anticipation that goes with building up to a delicious meal or your breakfast, say.

Remember how it feels to be hungry?

I had forgotten until I started this diet. I often ate because I was thirsty or bored, and had totally lost touch with the basics of appetite or enjoying the anticipation before sitting down to eat.

The first days of fasting were a revelation - because I realised I could feel hungry, acknowledge it, and then carry on with my day-to-day life. I would distract myself with sparkling water, black coffee or herbal tea, or even exercise. The pangs came in bursts and if I could ignore those, then they'd subside.

The key to being able to ignore those nagging hunger pangs? I knew it would be different the next day. I knew that if I couldn't put off eating what I fancied just for a few more hours until the next day (and knowing all the benefits to my body), then really there was no hope for me at all.

Willpower deserts me when a diet is never-ending. But when it's simply a matter of anticipating and enjoying my food the next day, it's so much easier.

Many others agree that soon the 'restriction' of a Fast Day begins to feel more like a 'liberation' from worrying about food – and allows the rest of your life to feel normal.

It allows me to have my Saturday night meal out and a few glasses of wine on a Friday without feeling as though I have 'broken my diet'. This means my relationship with my husband doesn't have to change, as we always eat out on Saturdays.

Julie 45

Fat Crimes and Punishments

The problem with previous diets has been the feeling of deprivation - even punishment that constant calorie counting can provoke. You start with the best of intentions but soon feel as though your newly restricted food intake is the penalty for being greedy. Then, in a difficult moment, you think 'sod it, if I'm greedy then so be it' and console yourself with the comfort food of choice - chocolate, cheese, bread, wine - which triggers a whole new cycle of guilt...

The issue with routines such as low-carbing, which require you to cut out most of an entire food group, is that it means you may never be able to enjoy the things you love - you see cake as sinful, or begin to fantasise about bread to go with your soup. Plus you gain a reputation as the picky one at friends' dinner parties or celebrations, which highlights the fact you're on a diet 'again' and also highlights any failures.

This diet changes how you view your eating habits. I see my Fast Days as a mini-break for my body, not to mention a break from cooking, as I tend to minimise the time in the kitchen. It's a reminder that there's more to life than food – it takes a few Fast Days to get used to that, but for me, it's liberating.

> *When you feel like you just HAVE to have something to eat, as hard as it may seem, just remember how bloated some foods make you, or the time you overindulged and felt bad, and remember how your body is using this 'fast' time to do really good things like healing and cleansing, and by the time you've remembered all of that you won't feel hungry again and it gets easier and easier to do.*
>
> Zoe, 38

Anita has been restricting her diet to shakes for the first two weeks, something that has worked really well for her.

> *Although the milkshakes were boring, I can see the benefit and pleased I took that route to start. a) I didn't have to think about calories on restricted days, therefore, I didn't think about food. b) Because the milkshake was so restricting, choosing*

what to eat after the two weeks were up,
has made me more aware of not to go over
my calorie limit – and I don't want to.

I've talked elsewhere about how hunger is no longer
something that scares me – and this diet is also teaching
me to enjoy my food more on both Fast and Feast Days –
my taste buds come alive and I enjoy every mouthful.

Without wishing to sound too precious, I am also
more *grateful* for the food I eat. Knowing that I can eat if I
really need to if the hunger becomes too great makes me
feel lucky that I have that choice, when so many people
don't.

The psychological benefits are one thing – but there
also seem to be benefits at cellular level, in terms of brain
function.

Effects on the brain: sharper, for longer?

The 'Horizon' TV programme introduced us to a rather
special breed of mouse. One that had been bred to develop
Alzheimer's disease. Different groups of these mice were
then fed different diets – some the equivalent of junk food,
others as much normal food as they wanted, and then
another group were subject to 'intermittent energy
restriction' – a day on/day off regime similar to ADF.

The last group were much slower to develop Alzheimer's even though they were destined to do so – and tests showed that the mice benefited from a range of changes including an increase in levels of <u>BDNF</u>, a protein that helps to protect existing neurons (brain cells) and encourage the growth of new ones. The mice on the ADF style regime also had better memories.

Why would fasting help the brain?

But why would this be happening? Again, common sense suggests that on reduced calories, the brain would be slowing down its activity, as the cells of the body do, rather than 'wasting' energy.

Neuroscientist Mark Mattson, from the American National Institute on Aging believes there's a biological reason why fasting would make the brain function better: if early man couldn't find or catch food, he'd go hungry and, ultimately, die. Therefore it makes absolute sense that his brain should work harder to either discover new sources of food or remember where he found it the last time.

So, fasting stresses the nerve cells but - as we've seen with the other medical research - this stress may be good stress, improving mental fitness, just as exercise stresses the muscles to improve physical fitness.

The research has implications not only for Alzheimer's (bit.ly/V5ewTv) and other forms of dementia, but also strokes (fxn.ws/Wx09q8). Mattson is now planning more research in humans to see whether fasting can stave off age-related cognitive decline. There are indications that the greatest benefits start at middle-age, so it may be that beginning this way of eating before that stage of life has less significant results.

You may also want to read this link, bit.ly/QPanph from a fasting advocate who examines some of the evidence for improvements in brain function, and other potential advantages of fasting. It makes very interesting reading.

For now, the human evidence isn't clear cut – but there's enough that Mattson has himself reportedly switched from a calorie restriction diet to intermittent fasting... I always think it's interesting to ask the experts how *they* eat.

To sum up:

So – 5:2 and other intermittent fasting or restriction diets can:

- Save you money
- Help you lose weight with minimal hassle
- Make it easier to maintain a healthy weight

And they may:

- Reduce your chances of developing life-threatening

diseases

- Change your attitude to food and hunger
- Help you stay mentally sharper, for longer

In the next part of the book, I'll explain how to adapt this diet so it works best for you. But first, will winter sun be my diet undoing?

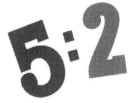

Hiccups in the sun

Mood: evangelical, positive, flexible

Everyone I talk to seems to know someone who is doing this diet - and it's as appealing to men as to women. I've been chatting to men about why, especially as so many men I know are reluctant to admit to dieting. Is it the all or nothing nature of the Fast Days? The simplicity of it? Or maybe it's just that it *really* works?

I've set up a page on Facebook called The 5:2 Diet so we can share our experiences. But the Facebook group is only the start - I feel so evangelical about this plan that I've decided to write all I know about it as an e-book - the book I wish there'd been when I first heard about it. I'm learning a lot by talking to others who are doing it.

The hiccups

Of course, the moment I decide to write
about the diet, my weight loss stalls. I
lose nothing in the first week and feel
slightly disheartened. There's a second
hiccup on the horizon. I'm off on holiday
to Tenerife for a week this month and I
know I won't be fasting there, so I decide
on a pre-emptive strike, switching to ADF -
fasting every other day - for the week
beforehand.

Again, I'm surprised how easy it is. I
simply fall into a routine of eating well
but unrestrictedly one day, and then being
extra careful the next. I hardly weigh any
foods out anymore but am grateful for
'gourmet' fresh soups… I know how cheap it
is to make your own, but it also involves
being tempted to add little extras to the
recipe, whereas these pots involve no more
preparation than pressing a button on the
microwave.

Cheap as Chips

On top of this, I'm also saving money through this diet - cutting back on my snacking on Fast Days, but also on Feast Days because I am somehow more able to ask myself the question: do I really want this? If I do, then it's absolutely fine. But even being able to ask that question seems to curb my appetite.

And on the Fast Days I am eating very little, so my shopping bill is going down - unlike when I was low-carbing, and had to buy lots of expensive protein - or when I was doing normal calorie counting and spent a fair amount on special 'low-cal' options which always cost more.

There are occasional comedy moments, too - like the day I took a chip off my boyfriend's plate, then insisted on weighing a similar-sized one and entering it into MyFitnessPal. One chip = 8 calories = too much!

A week off-piste

I didn't count a single calorie on holiday.
Buffet breakfasts, buffet dinners and lots
of lovely Spanish wine. Buffets are
notorious with diet researchers, as the
variety makes us go a bit crazy, grabbing a
little bit of this and that and the other
which adds up to far more calories than
we'd eat at a normal meal. But I am more
conscious of stopping when I am hungry, not
least because my bikini body is still not
quite what I'd like it to be.

With that in mind I do something
unprecedented - go the hotel gym!
Fourtimes. It's not easy because the
weather is hot and the gym's not air-
conditioned and the equipment is pretty
basic, but I do it. Everyone else in the
gym is very buff and I feel like I stand
out a bit but, could it be possible that I
am turning into one of *those* people?

Back to Fasting and Feasting

I loved my holiday but I am also looking
forward to coming back to my food routine.

I like the thought it's doing me good as well as making me look better in my clothes. I stick with ADF - roughly, it's probably more like three Fast Days a week - and deliberately don't weigh myself in the week or so after I return from holidays because I don't want to feel down-hearted. But my jeans are still looser than they were.

My routine is pretty fixed now, but I'm experimenting with exercise. I did join the gym just before I started this lifestyle but it's become more important to me while I'm doing this - at first, I avoided exercising on a Fast Day but recently I've tried it and it's fine for me. I don't feel noticeably dizzy or wobbly if I do it. And the exercise just feels like part of what I want to do to look after myself more, and maximise the benefits of the diet.

The Eggs Florentine Episode

The one thing with this way of eating is that it can be slightly less sociable. It's easy to schedule the diet for a couple of days a week when you have nothing planned, but Alternate Day Fasting inevitably involves a weekend day, and that's bound to be the one that happens to coincide with a spontaneous brunch. Which is what happened on Sunday. We went to my favourite cafe - Temptation in Brighton, you *have* to go if you're in town - and I'd thought, that's fine, I'll have the soup.

Then came the bombshell - they don't serve soup at weekends!

There was nothing on the menu that seemed likely to be under 500 calories. Their breakfasts are legendary, their cakes towering, and I was grumpy as I ordered black coffee and braced myself to watch everyone else scoffing breakfast.

'This is very anti-social,' said the boyfriend. 'And perhaps a little obsessive. After all, it's only one day. One meal.'

I tried to think about the counterarguments - the fact that the Fast Days do involve commitment. And yet...

I ordered the eggs Florentine: two poached eggs, spinach, sourdough toast and - this is the only unhealthy bit - lashings of sunshine yellow hollandaise sauce, vowing that I'd scrape off the sauce, even though it's my favourite bit.

And then I scoffed the lot.

At home, I looked up Hollandaise on MyFitnessPal. When I've tried to make it myself, it involved vast quantities of butter. So yes, it was high fat and very calorific. But so what if I'd gone over on one of my Fast Days? It's one day in my life. What this diet is doing is making me aware and informed about what I put in my body.

The Eggs Florentine Episode is a warning not to take it *too* seriously. To live a little.

And, guess what? I didn't actually feel hungry for the rest of the day...

Weight on October 31st: 150lbs: total lost 11lbs

Days on diet: 83

BMI 25.9 - which means I'm within a point of a healthy BMI

OK, it's only a loss of two pounds this month but I have had a great holiday, plus I think I am putting on muscle from the gym.

As for my goal - well, till now I haven't dared have one, but I think I'd like to be a nice round (well, not *that* round) 10 stone (63.5 kg) - or maybe 9 stone 13 (63 kg) to be in single figures.

Watch this space...

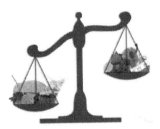

Part Two: 5:2 Your Way

Planning and personalising for success

Step One: How much do you want to lose, and how much can you afford to eat?

A lot of this chapter is about sums. Sorry.

Of course, weight loss shouldn't only be about numbers - it's about how you feel, and look, and how well the body's working - but if you want to fine-tune the diet then there is a small amount of counting to be done at first. The good news is that it should take you no time at all to work the figures out, and once you have, you're all set.

Goal setting: where do you want to be?

Weigh yourself
Yes, I know. It's grim. But the good thing about weighing yourself is that in no time you'll be feeling smug when you're losing weight. If you've knocked a few pounds off now, because you hate what you see on the scales, your weight loss won't show up....

Calculate your BMI
As I've said elsewhere, BMI isn't always the best indicator of your weight level, especially if you're very athletic, but it does give a basic indicator. You calculate it using this simple formula –

BMI = Weight (kg) / [Height (m) x Height (m)]

Or - even more simply - by using the calculators on MyFitnessPal.com or other weight loss sites (just search for BMI calculator).

Work out now whether you want your target weight loss to be measured in BMI goals e.g. a BMI of 24, or in the equivalent weight in pounds or kg. So, for example for me, my goal weight is 9 stone 13, which is a) in single figures when it comes to stones, just (!) and b) represents a BMI of 23.83...

If you're doing 5:2 for the health benefits, it still makes sense to track your weight - you don't want to slip into the underweight category as that too can have health implications. If you monitor it, you can make adjustments, e.g. moving to 6:1 with just one fasting day a week.

Diet calculations: how to reach your goal?

How many days a week can you fast/calorie restrict?

The diet is called 5:2 by many people because the ratio of 5 'normal' days and 2 'diet' days works really well for most people - it does seem to guarantee some weight loss, but it's manageable in terms of finding quieter days when it works to eat less, and also means you don't feel like you're on a diet most of the time.

Our dieters have made a variety of choices:

> *I follow standard 5:2, but probably consume 7-800 calories on fast days (but I'm tall and exercise a lot) .*
>
> *James, 43*
>
> *2 days, 500 cals and I don't do breakfast now.*
>
> *Julia, 50*
>
> *Every other day - 500 calories.*
>
> *Sally, 49*
>
> *Two days and I aim for about 600 calories a day as I don't need to lose weight.*
>
> *Nina, 52*
>
> *Two days. 300 calories.*
>
> *Sarah, 37*

Many people also do 4:3 (3 days of restriction) or Alternate Day Fasting (ADF) where you'll do the diet every other day, which ensures a more rapid weight loss. For those mainly seeking the health benefits, without weight loss, 6:1 seems to be the preferred option.

How much should you eat on this diet?

Fast Days (the 2 in the 5:2 diet) are when you are restricting your calorie intake to approximately 25% of your daily calorific requirement (DCR).

You can either calculate your exact DCR using the method outlined below,

OR

If the idea of any more sums makes you queasy, you can work on averages.

The average active woman needs approximately 2000 calories per day (or what we know of as calories: most food labels list kcals or kilo calories but 'calories' is used interchangeably in most diet books, including this one. So your goal intake for Fast Days is 500.

Active men need on average 2400 calories a day so they get an extra 100 cals or a goal intake of 600 calories.

Want to do it the proper way? Calculating your personal goal is a three-stage, ABC process.

Stage A: what a girl (or guy) needs

You begin by working out the Basal Metabolic Rate - that's an estimate of how many calories someone of your size, height and age might need just to get through the day. That is, to keep your most basic functions going. There are two different formulas as well (the Harris Benedict and the Mifflin St Jeor version.

Harris Benedict:
Male = (13.75 x w) + (5 x h) - (6.76 x a) + 66
Female = (9.56 x w) + (1.85 x h) - (4.68 x a) + 655

Mifflin St Jeor:
Male: BMR = 10×weight + 6.25×height - 5×age + 5
Female: BMR = 10×weight + 6.25×height - 5×age - 161

Too much maths for me. It's much easier to use an online calculator via www.myfitnesspal.com/tools instead. Again, you can choose whichever you prefer, but remember which you've used for future reference, as you will want to recalculate when or if your weight or activity level changes.

Let's take the example of a fifty-year-old man, 5 feet 10 tall, and weighing 14 stone (196 pounds).

Estimated BMR: 1755 calories per day

Stage B: higher, higher!

Remember, the BMR is just about your most basic needs - you take that figure and apply another calculation based on how active you are, to give you a truer estimate of your actual requirements. This involves multiplying the BMR from Step A by a number determined by how much exercise you do.

Little/no exercise: BMR x 1.2 = Total Calorie Need
Light exercise: BMR x 1.375 = Total Calorie Need
Moderate exercise (3-5 days/wk): BMR x 1.55 = Total Calorie Need
Very active (6-7 days/wk): BMR x 1.725 = Total Calorie Need
Extra active (very active & physical job): BMR x 1.9 = Total Calorie Need

Our male dieter takes limited light exercise, so we multiply his BMR by 1.375:

1755 x 1.55 = 2413 calories

This is an estimate of the number of calories he should consume each day to maintain his current weight – the DCR - daily calorie requirement.

Stage C: Lower, lower!

To count as a fast - and potentially bring a dieter all the health benefits that scientists are researching - it's understood that you should aim to eat a quarter or 25% of your DCR figure on Fast Days.

So in our example, we need to multiply the DCR by 0.25:

$$2413 \times 0.24 = 603 \text{ calories}$$

In this case, the limit is pretty close to the 600 for men that Dr Mosley recommended for his programme – but do note that this would change if our example were less active, or as he loses weight. It's why you'll want to recalculate as you go along, perhaps with every seven pounds you lose? Alas, as you lose weight, your calorie requirement decreases – UNLESS you step up your levels of activity, which may well happen as you find you have more energy and confidence.

So that's the sums done. I promised you the most flexible diet you've ever tried - so it's time to tailor the diet to suit you!

Which day(s) do I fast?

Picking the right days will improve your chances of success, especially to begin with.

The first time(s) you fast, you're likely to feel hungry at first, with possible other side-effects like headaches, or feeling cold or slightly light-headed. Most of us become used to this very quickly, but it makes sense to schedule your first Fast Days for the days of the week when you have fewer commitments and can afford to take it a little easier. It's the same with most diets but with this one, it's important - even more so if you're driving, operating machinery, caring for others or involved in a high-stress or high-risk occupation.

Choose days when you have no social engagements, or don't have to be around people who might be sceptical or try to persuade you to give up. If you are responsible for family meals, then try to build in days when the meal is healthier and you can have a small portion without attracting too much fuss. I like to do my Fast Days when my partner is working late or socialising with friends because that way I won't be tempted to eat what he's eating at home!

It's good to have regular days if you can, e.g. Monday and Wednesday, because you can then schedule around it - I now exercise on Fast Days but I didn't feel able to do that at first, so it can be much easier to schedule a fitness class or a long walk on Feast Days. But it's your diet - feel free to experiment.

I definitely find it helps to mark the Fast Days on my e-calendar and to-do lists – this way I feel that I have committed to them!

WHEN will I eat on my Fast Days?

You can choose to eat your calorie allowance in one, two or even three meals, although some evidence suggests that it's better to restrict to one or two and this is how Krista Varady's study worked: with participants having a single, larger meal at lunchtime on their 'fast' days. This makes sense to me because it appears to give the body less to 'do' in terms of digesting food, producing insulin etc. Dr Mosley, by contrast, decided that he would eat two meals and it still worked for him, both in terms of weight loss and reduction in IGF-1.

That's the beauty of this diet compared to all the others I've tried (and abandoned): you decide how to make the diet fit your life, rather than the diet dictating how to live it.

> *No breakfast. Porridge midday. Veg soup in evening. Couple of barley cups during day and perhaps a rice cake.*
>
> Stephen, 47

One meal in the evening with my family. Portions small except for green salad/veg. An entire bag of salad is circa 40 calories (a single egg is circa 80 calories and as for cheese or, god forbid mayonnaise...!)

Myfanwy, 49

I can't do just one meal a day as I need the psychological feeling of having three meals a day.

Nina, 52

I'm afraid I haven't got to the stage of fasting all day, but at the moment spread my 500 over 8 hours.

Claire, 43

One evening meal - usually a bowl of soup, or a plate of vegetables. I'm not very exact.

Sarah, 37

Many 5:2 and ADF dieters also like to try to maximise the gap between the last meal on Feast Day and the Fast Day, and also between the last meal on the Fast Day and the first meal on the following Feast Day. For example:

Monday Feast Day:
　　Eat dinner at 6pm

Tuesday Fast Day:

   Eat main meal at 6pm (no breakfast or lunch)

Wednesday Feast Day:

        Skip breakfast, eat lunch late e.g. 2pm

Again, there's no indisputable evidence on whether this works better, but I try to maximise the gaps for the same reasons, that I sense it gives my body a rest from digesting/processing foods.

Maximising the benefits: the full Fast Day?

Some 5:2 dieters do decide to try a 'full' fast, where you only drink water or herbal teas: using this method you could manage to fast for 44 hours, yet there's only one day where you can't actually eat the food you enjoy.

This is how it would look:

Monday Feast Day:

                Eat dinner at 6pm

Tuesday Fast Day:

                Fast completely

Wednesday Feast Day:

        Skip breakfast, eat lunch late e.g. 2pm

If that sounds a bit hard-core to you, don't worry. But it might be something for the future. It would certainly have seemed too daunting for me before I began the 5:2 diet, but now I might try it in the new year as a good reintroduction to the diet.

There are plenty of other versions of fasting diets talked about online and on forums: if you join one of the groups in the resources section, you can find out more about what other people are trying.

Bear in mind that total fasts can be harder to stick to, but there are many alternatives, such as compressing your mealtimes into a small 'window', so you avoid food for twenty hours and limit eating to between , say, 1pm and 5pm.

I try to postpone eating all day so I can eat in the evenings but I'm not sure this helps much. It probably does re: the metabolic changes needed for fat mobilisation and brain growth, because the longer we go, the better it is, but it might undermine the repair at night side of things. The research suggested eating at mid-day but I fear once I start eating I would want more.

Linda, 52

The truth is that there isn't enough evidence yet about what precise configuration of fasting will work best. So turn that to your advantage: experiment and see which works for you within your daily routine.

Consecutive or non-consecutive?

Most people find it easier to schedule the days non-consecutively as the hunger pangs can be stronger and a two-day fast can become an ordeal rather than a 'mini-break'. This risks making it less sustainable than the non-consecutive option. Also, fasting for two days may increase the risk of Starvation Mode, which we don't want (see Chapter Three).

WHAT will I eat on my Fast Day?

Exactly what you like... so long as it doesn't exceed your calorie limit.

500 or 600 calories isn't a lot to play with. But, take it from me, you *can* still make satisfying choices.

Banana for breakfast. Apple and yoghurt for lunch. Chicken and salad for dinner.

Karl, 49

Loads of cups of tea with a little milk, nothing till supper, then a normal family supper with few/no carbs.

Julia, 50

Only water!

Rob, 42

All home-made food so it's hard to work out the calories. I'll avoid carbs and alcohol and have a small helping of chicken or fish and lots of vegetables - a bowl of home-made soup and fruit for the other meal. I'm aiming to only eat between 12 and 6, too, on most other days.

Linda, 52

I stick to fruit and veg, beans on toast, soups, Weight Watcher ready meals.

Jane, 49

There are **two** fundamental choices with this diet:

    EITHER, regard it as a break from worrying too much about cooking and food preparation, and focus on ready-made dishes or simply-cooked vegetables and proteins;

    OR, see it as a challenge to make home-cooked food with as low a calorie count as possible.

I must confess I started with the latter approach but tend now towards the former - the less time in the kitchen, the fewer the temptations. But there are lots of suggestions in Part Three for both approaches. However you choose to do it, I do recommend planning in advance - the very last thing you want to be doing on your first Fast Day is going into the supermarket...

Obviously, it also depends on how many meals you're planning to have - it's very easy to find ready-meals with 400-500 calories if you're only having a single meal, but it gets slightly harder if you want two or even three. That's where soups come into play - they tend to fill you up for longer, with fewer calories.

I am also more careful to remember to take a multi-vitamin during the fasts: not because I think a day or two of eating less will do serious damage, but it's a good insurance policy.

HOW will I monitor my consumption?

Studies suggest that dieters who keep a record of their consumption tend to be more successful, and it will help you pinpoint where you might be going wrong if you need to amend your habits or consumption.

If you're going for ready-made meals, recording your consumption can be very easy - just read the nutritional information on the packet and either write down the totals or use MyFitnessPal or similar apps/sites to record what you eat. You can keep your diary completely private or, if you find it helps to keep you motivated, share it with others.

If you are using ingredients or creating 'doll's house portions' of regular meals, then I recommend investing in a digital/electronic scale as it will measure to the last gram - very handy when you're trying to calculate how many calories in a single, lusted-after tortilla chip. You can then either calculate the calories via MyFitnessPal, or using a simple calorie counter book. I prefer MyFitnessPal because it does the sums for you *and* thousands of other users are constantly updating the site with new foods or brands. On top of this, you can use it to calorie-count your own recipes. It's how I've done the dishes in Part Three, for example.

At first, you'll probably be astonished at how such a tiny portion can weigh so much - but after a while you'll be able to ease off with familiar ingredients. A cheaper alternative to a scale would be measuring spoons but be careful not to overload them!

That's enough theory... are you ready to try your first fast?

Step Two: Your First Fast

It's here... your first Fast Day.

If you've followed the guidance in the last section, you'll be ready for anything. You will know how much to eat, and be ready to experiment with when and what. So this section is mainly about strategies and tips from those of us who have been there...

Motivation

The biggest motivation for many of us has been the maxim:

It's only a day – tomorrow you can eat what you feel like!

But here are some more tips straight from the 5:2 dieters' mouths:

> *Have a plan for the week and measure out what 500 calories looks like. This will stop you obsessing about food ALL day long. Thinking of what you will reward yourself with is also good. I plan to have a nice Thai meal with all those 'naughty' carbs.*

> *Zoe 38*

Try to leave breakfast as late as possible. When you eat in the morning it makes you feel like you want to eat more. I prefer to leave my meals as late as I can. For snacking, try cherry tomatoes or carrots. Not many calories but filling. I prefer getting the fast days over and done early in the week - Mondays and Wednesdays. Fasting on days when you are not at work is harder as you have more temptations around.

Sunil, 34

Find something to keep you busy well away from food (I fast on work days, if I can; hardly have time to eat there anyway) and treat yourself on non-fasting days so you don't feel deprived.

Myfanwy, 49

Drink lots of boiled water or herbal teas on your fasting day. Every time you feel peckish, have a herbal tea and you'll find the flavour makes you feel as if you've eaten something. Also, if you like milk in your tea or coffee first thing in the morning and last thing at night, have it, even on fasting day. There's no need to count it amongst your calories and it won't do you any harm. It will make you feel less as if you're being punished for something. It also helps to choose one treat that you intend to have the next day when you can eat what you want again, whether it's a bit of cake, some chocolate, a glass of wine, or a full English breakfast.

Sally, 49

Finally, I love this cautionary tale from Myfanwy:

DON'T go food shopping on a Fast Day - last time I did I came home with a turkey (on special offer). Admittedly it was a runt of a turkey but I don't even like turkey and I've never cooked one before in my life. The family thought it was hilarious.

Myfanwy, 49

Friends and Frenemies:

One question which does crop up is, *Who should I tell?*

Obviously, if you know friends or family members who are already on the diet, then they will be sympathetic

136

– but some of our dieters were surprised at people's reactions:

> *I find it embarrassing being on a fasting diet (because I know people will exclaim 'you're too thin to be doing it) so I don't talk about it outside our family. If I'm ever with other people on fasting days I tend to try and eat as little as possible without people noticing.*
>
> Sarah, 37

> *I told a few people I was starting the fast and it both helped & hindered me. It helped because when I was a little cranky on those first couple of fasts they just took it as the diet, but it hindered because any conversation I had where we didn't agree (not an argument, just work related or otherwise) they said I wasn't being rational because I 'needed to eat something' which wasn't the case as both times I had just eaten and they were not 'fast' days! Be prepared for doubters as most people are 'brainwashed' about 'skipping meals' and 'breakfast is the most important meal of the*

day' and 'your metabolism will slow down' so I don't talk about the diet anymore, I just get on with it.

Zoe, 38

Men in particular can find it embarrassing to be on an obvious diet – one recent survey suggested one in three male dieters wouldn't admit it, even to their closest friends or family. Though our group of software company employees have definitely seen the benefits of sharing:

If a group of you are doing it, it really helps – especially if you all do it on the same day.

Andrew, 42

But even if you can't or don't want to get colleagues involved, the internet makes it really easy to connect with diet soul mates. Joining in with a forum can really help – because we can talk online to people who have been there and ask questions without feeling embarrassed: there are plenty of forums listed in the Resources section of this book.

You may also worry about the impression a fasting diet might give to younger people in your family, especially now there's so much more awareness around eating disorders.

I have three daughters and I am concerned about setting a good example, and not making them too faddy. So when they're around I stick to something simple, like beans on toast, which doesn't look like a 'fasting' meal.

Mary, 50

Practical Tips:

o It's worth re-reading Chapters Three and Four about the potential health benefits before or after a Fast Day to remind yourself that you're doing something that's about more than vanity.

o If you can, avoid situations where you have to watch other people eat – or have to cook for the family. If you can't get out of doing the cooking, choose Fast Days to cook the things you really don't like and they do!

o Sugar-free chewing gum is another standby!

o Evenings can be a dangerous time for snackers - a hobby that uses your hands (quiet at the back!) like knitting, sewing, even jigsaws, can keep you from raiding the biscuit barrel when you're watching TV.

o Don't forget to drink water! As well as eating up to your goal calorie limit, you can (and should) drink plenty of water – there's evidence that good hydration helps with fat loss.

- o I like to drink sparkling water on Fast Days – somehow it's more enjoyable!
- o You may also drink black coffee or tea, herb teas and diet drinks, although artificially sweetened drinks may still affect your blood sugar or insulin levels, which is not ideal on a Fast Day. There is also some debate about the effect that caffeine has on insulin – with some studies showing an increase in insulin sensitivity (which would be broadly good news) and others showing insulin spikes (less good news). As an espresso addict, I am sticking with my daily fixes for now but as with all the decisions here, it's about personal choice.
- o You may feel like going to bed early on the first few Fast Days – so use it as an excuse to relax!

And **REMEMBER:**

Tomorrow you can eat what you like!

The positives about Fast Days:
- o Knowing you're doing something good for your health and your body
- o Reminding yourself what hungry feels like - it's

a useful thing to know because it stops you confusing it with boredom or thirst, say, when you're on a normal eating day

o   Realising you can work past hunger - after an hour or so, provided you have no other health problems, any pangs will often reduce

o   Mindfulness and gratefulness for the food you *can* eat, and also for the fact that when the fast is over you can eat what you like

o   Not to mention the fact that any food you do have scheduled will be savoured all the more!

o   It can be a break for your mind *and* body as you focus on things other than food - though that may not kick in till you've done a few fasts

The possible side-effects

You may not experience any of these, but here are some of the more common things dieters have experienced in the early days. Jeanny is typical:

> *I have been feeling light headed and dizzy, but I'm not sure whether it is the diet as I haven't been doing it very long yet. Also, have had several headaches.*

> *Jeanny, 53*

Trouble-shooting any unwelcome symptoms:

- Headaches - keeping liquid levels up can be useful here. Also, varying the times you eat may reduce this.

- Feeling cold - especially in winter. I'm not sure if this is physical, mental or a combination, but hot drinks and eating soup do help. Also try adding spices to foods, like flaked chilli. This works wonders with soup or baked beans...

- Irritability - it's a natural response to feeling hungry but this will abate once you have become used to the sensation. Try one of the lower-calorie treats in the food section – it's better to do without them in the long-term, but when you're starting out try whatever gets you through!

- Digestive changes: constipation, reflux - these have been reported by some 5:2 people – it's worth including fibre (e.g. baked beans) or 'digestive transit' yogurts in your Fast Days. One of our dieters was advised by her surgery nurse to ask the pharmacist about gentle laxatives, though obviously these are not recommended for anything other than occasional use.

- Cramps - I used to get these all the time on low-carb diets and haven't on this one. But I know some people have and I've read about good responses to potassium, magnesium or calcium supplements (read more at bit.ly/TsrDvY).

Ready, steady, fast....

And that's all there is to it.

By the end of today, you'll have finished your first fast - the first, we hope, of many that will help you keep a check on your eating and improve your health.

Step Three: Review, Revise, Revitalise

The Day After

You did it! And today you can enjoy the foods you love - perhaps some of the things you were craving yesterday... what are you most looking forward to?

We've talked a lot about Fast Days – but what about Feast Days? These are times to relax and enjoy food and all the great things around food – being with friends and family, savouring the tastes and smells and pleasure of cooking or eating out. In fact, it's not *just* about the food.

> *I find that I sleep much deeper on starving nights and wake up feeling more fresh than normal. Also, the sun seems brighter, the sky bluer and the song of birds more beautiful on the day after starving. ;)*
>
> Sunil, 34

On Feast Days you can eat 'normally' – but what does that actually mean? One of the things I've discovered since starting this lifestyle is that I did eat much more than I realised. So while my own 'doll's house portions' on Fast Days seem ludicrously small, the portions served in restaurants now often seem obscenely super-sized.

For me, the view of what a 'portion' of food is has become skewed and that's one of the reasons many of us have suffered weight problems. So, although you can eat all the things you love on your normal days, there's clearly a sensible balance. This diet will probably re-educate you by stealth. You'll become fuller sooner, and you'll enjoy your favourite foods but perhaps not in the same quantities. Bear in mind that you are still aiming for that calorie deficit we discussed in Chapter Two: most people don't need to calorie count to achieve that.

The work done by Krista Varady at the University of Illinois compared alternate day fasters who ate a low-fat diet on their feast day, with those who ate a 'normal' high-fat diet when they weren't fasting. Surprisingly – and happily – the reduction in weight and cholesterol was as good, if not better, in those participants who were encouraged to eat all their favourite dishes, including pizza and burgers.

It's a finding backed up by the software engineers who've clubbed together to track their experiences on 5:2.

We have seen no difference in effect if you eat high fat or low fat food on non-fasting days. In fact, where some of us have been away on holiday, we have temporarily stopped and then restarted with little overall effect.

Andrew, 42

Of course, what you eat is one thing. How much is another matter. I admit that in the first week or two, I was tempted to over-eat the things I loved. But that soon wore off, as it has for other 5:2 dieters. Even eating your Daily Calorie Requirement (DCR) - just under 2000 calories in my case - feels like such a feast compared to the fasting that you probably won't feel the need to exceed it and, on many occasions, you'll eat less than you used to.

Mindful Eating

One tip while you're adapting would be to use the same tactic many of us use on the Fast Days - to eat very slowly, with no other distractions. So, no TV, work or multi-tasking. Savouring your food rather than throwing it down means you'll probably be less tempted to overeat. But you certainly don't need to record what you're eating on the Feast Days.

Mindfulness – a form of meditation – can be a very useful tool in both controlling appetite and feeling positive and calm about the changes you're making. A friend recommended the getsomeheadspace.com site, which offers a free introductory trial of meditations, as well as some really useful downloads, including one on mindful eating (bit.ly/QPbKEh). Or read more about other people's experiences in *The Independent* (ind.pn/QsEwJp) and *The*

New York Times (nyti.ms/U4Fis5). You'll find it easier to follow these links via the list downloadable for free from my site at kate-harrison.com/52diet

What if I'm not losing enough weight?

If, a few weeks down the line, you're not losing as much weight as you hope, it might be advisable to use MyFitnessPal or a calorie counting book to double-check your calorie consumption on a couple of Feast Days. Obviously, as we saw in Chapter Two, fasting will cut anything from 3,000 to 6,000 calories from your weekly consumption, but if you do find you are bingeing or over-compensating, then the weight loss could stall.

Be aware of what you're eating if you are stuck – or perhaps consider fasting on Alternate Days for a week or two to speed things along?

The good news is that most people find the Fast and Feast pattern helps them find a natural balance of enjoying food without overindulging.

It gets easier!

If you find your Fast Day tough, then take comfort from the fact that most of us have found they get easier – much easier. Whether it's because we become used to less food, or our stomachs shrink, is unclear.

But it definitely becomes less of a chore, and many dieters report a feeling of lightness and euphoria on Fast Days – feeling good physically, but also psychologically, knowing that you're doing something good for your body, not simply depriving it.

Reviewing and Planning your Next Fasts

The first few weeks are about experimenting with what works for you - the best mealtimes, the most satisfying foods, plus any hints to reduce any side-effects you might be feeling.

Get into the habit of planning the days you'll be fasting the next week, and preparing by buying any ready meals, or the ingredients for home-made dishes. Check the food section of this book for more ideas and options.

Are you someone who craves variety or a person who will be happy with the same foods on your Fast Day? I've mentioned my huge beetroot-fest that lasted or about a month during the diet, without any side effects. Then gradually, and naturally, I switched to something else. If the idea of eating the same thing on Fast Days will damage your motivation, then experiment and go onto forums to check out what ideas people have, especially for eating seasonally (which is also likely to be cheaper!).

Exercise and 5:2

I've suggested that at first you avoid exercise during Fast Days - until you know how your body reacts to the calorie restriction.

I started doing my gym visits on Fast Days about a month after I began the diet. At first, I did feel light-headed at times, and reduced the pace a little, but I've found that I can now keep up the exercise intensity on Fast and Feast Days.

Here's what other dieters have to say:

> *I typically jog 6km 4 times a week. It makes no different if that is a diet day.*
>
> *Stephen, 47*

> *On fasting days I do thirty minutes on the treadmill at 2mph. As I have arthritis at the moment this is the most I can do without bringing on an 'episode' of arthritis, but I hope to build it up as I lose weight/get fitter. I try to do this every day but if I feel sore I will rest for a day or two.*
>
> *Sally, 49*

I haven't found it easy to exercise on Fast Days, but on other days I will spend two to three evenings a week in the gym doing weights, cardio and swimming.

Claire, 43

I work 5 days per week, long hours in a sit-down job. Walking is my main exercise which I try to do often, and always for at least an hour and a half on Saturday and Sunday (dog walking)!

Steph, 49

I've maintained my usual routine of daily exercise (mostly cycling to work). I generally avoid tough workouts on fasting days.

James, 43

So much for my good intentions. I don't go to the gym but I have tried to walk more. On Fast Days this will be quite effective in increasing the energy deficit. On non-Fast Days it's just good for me.

Linda, 52

I run about four times a week – thirty mins each time. It doesn't really matter if I do it on Fast or Non Fast Days because it doesn't increase my appetite. I don't factor it into my calorie restriction because I don't think it makes that much difference.

Sarah, 37

There's a debate about whether exercising on Fast Days, or on an empty stomach before breakfast, for example, might have benefits (bit.ly/Tv2owD) although an analysis (bit.ly/Vgv6Uh) on the NHS website suggests that it's too early to draw conclusions. For now it's good to do what feels right for you but do be wary of pushing yourself too hard at first, and consult your doctor if you have any doubts at all.

Weighing In

Most diets recommend weighing yourself no more than once a week, because fluid levels and weight fluctuates so much, especially, for women, during the monthly menstrual cycle.

Opinions vary, of course:

One thing I'd warn against is weighing too often. I was tempted to weigh myself every day (and did!) when I started, but it can be a bit soul destroying as you'll find you'll lose weight on fasting days then appear to put it back on again on feasting days. It's best to weigh once a week.

Sally, 49

But another forum member thinks the opposite:

If you can bear it, weigh every day, fast and non-fast, because you can track what's happening and the pattern of losing weight. Provided you stick to it, it'll still be downwards...

Kevin, 40

For most of us, the best thing is to record it only once a week, either in a notebook or on a site like MyFitnessPal (which will later produce a nice graph for you, hopefully showing your excellent progress!).

I tend to weigh the morning after the second Fast Day of a week, first thing, before I've eaten. At first it felt like cheating but so long as you always do it at the same time, then the progress or otherwise will become clear.

Rewarding Yourself

Any lifestyle change can be tricky, and it makes sense to find ways to reward yourself in ways that don't involve food - the standard advice is things like a long hot bath, a massage, new clothes.

But if you're not into girly (or man) treats, or you haven't reached your goal weight, brainstorm other rewards - a new DVD box set or even a fitness DVD; a great novel; tickets for a gig or a gallery; whatever you love doing that you don't always give yourself time to enjoy.

You could put aside the money you're saving from your grocery bill to pay for the treats.

I have even been known to reward myself with a new recipe book, for the days when I can enjoy cooking without feeling guilty. There's pleasure in the gloriously illogical knowledge that weight loss is contributing to my next delicious meal on a Feast Day!

The Gift of Food

I'd like to share one story from forty-three-year-old Jenny, who is finding that her fasts are making her see the world differently, too.

It really is a very good way of eating (I don't call it a diet!) and have to say, on a

vaguely hippy level, I feel humbled by the fact that I can choose to go hungry. A homeless girl stopped me in the street the other day and asked if I could spare her a pound for a hot drink. I've never been approached directly like that before. But something in my brain pinged and I realised that I had chosen not to nip out of the office for a sarnie and pot of fruit since it was a fasting day. So I gave her the fiver I'd have spent on lunch. You'd think I'd given a wheelbarrow full of treasure. It's funny how things strike you at just the right time - homeless people are a factor in any big town or city yet being approached by that girl seems like proper synchronicity.

I realise I feel the same way as Jenny, and have decided to mark each seven pounds I lose on the diet with a donation to charity: a way of acknowledging how lucky I am to be able to choose to do this. If it's something that appeals to you, you might consider doing the same.

The Best Reward - it works...

Of course, you should soon begin seeing the results of the diet itself - which is the biggest reward. Many of us see changes from week one - mine wasn't dramatic from the start but it did feel very sustainable. And the reward of feeling more in control was an unexpected bonus.

Trouble-shooting

What if it's *not* working quite as you'd hoped? In a few cases, that might be the case.

- o Review your Feast Days - do a trial calorie count on one or two days. If it exceeds your DCR (Daily Calorific Requirement – see the calculations in Step One of the book) by a large amount you may need to adjust your portion sizes, which should be less daunting than it would have seemed before you began the diet.

- o There are a few people who stick to the diet but don't see the results. If you've done some calorie counting and you're not bingeing, it may be worth talking to your doctor about thyroid or other issues, especially if you've struggled on other diets too.

Now move onto Part Three - it's all about the food!

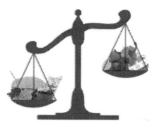

Part Three: Eating the 5:2 way

Home cooking or convenience foods – you choose!

Overview

There's no point in fibbing about this - you can't eat much on your Fast Days. But even 500-600 calories can fill you up, and for most of us, it's far less daunting than a 'true' fast where you'd eat nothing at all.

Here are a few daily menus from our 5:2 experts.

Usually have 100g frozen fruit for breakfast (thawed - 29 cals). Weight Watchers tomato soup (76 cals) at lunchtime and either a Weight Watchers frozen meal in the evening, or fish or chicken with salad in the evening to make up to the 500, less if possible. Allow 60 cals for 2 coffees with milk during the day. Weight Watchers chicken and beef hotpots are about 230 cals each.

Steph, 49

1x Coffee (white with sugar)
1x cup-a-soup for lunch
2 pieces of fruit in late afternoon
A decent meal in the evening

Also drink herbal teas during the day if I feel peckish

Shop-bought soups (as low-calorie as possible) and ready meals, with some veg and fruit. I aim for 500 calories and total it as I go.

Val, 56

*Oats So Simple Porridge with Semi-Skimmed Milk at around 1pm (180 calories)
Bachelors Golden Vegetable Cup-a-soup at around 4:30pm (59 calories)
Dinner usually around 300-350 calories, often from the Hairy Bikers Diet Cook Book which is excellent as it's not low fat and gives calories per portion.*

Andrew, 42

I've started making dhal, baked beans are good, salads are filling, make my own tom soup with a half stock cube in a little boiling water, 1/3rd tom puree added once that's dissolved, herbs and garlic puree added (the stuff in the tube), then topped up with more boiling water. Easy. I avoid hi GI foods.

Linda, 52

Yogurt, cuppa soup, and an omelette!

Graeme, 38

As I outlined in <u>Step Two</u>, you will need to make decisions about how often you eat on your Fast Day – one, two, or three meals - and also whether you want to cook, or use ready-made meals. Many of us do both, though as I carry on with this regime I veer more towards spending the minimum time in the kitchen. I adore cooking but it's less fun when you're measuring every teaspoon of vinegar, or fretting over lemon juice.

In this part of the book, I will make suggestions for ready-made *and* home-made options for breakfasts, lunches and dinners, plus snacks, treats and tips for eating out. Equally, if you want to munch on muesli at tea time, or sip soup for breakfast, of course it's your call!

The recipes are pretty simple and basic out of necessity - and remember you can alter them, or put your own dishes into the Recipe section of the www.MyFitnessPal.com site to work out how many calories your favourites contain. You can make a huge batch of soup or stew and then measure it out into portions to freeze –

this way you enjoy all the economic benefits of a home-made dish, but run less risk of accidentally going over the limit for the day.

I'm a vegetarian and I do recommend focusing on fruit and veg on your Fast Days as you'll get more for your calories - though there are meaty suggestions too.

Also bear in mind that some scientists say eating a lot of protein may switch on IGF-1 which may be counter-productive. Dr Mosley has said he tries to stick to 55g of protein on Fast Days – as an example, a medium egg contains approximately 7g and 100g of cooked chicken breast contains around 30g. You may prefer to keep protein levels down - it's a balance, though, as protein contains more calories but tends to keep you full for longer.

I've also included an A-Z (with a few letters missing, I must admit - ever tried finding a nice food beginning with U?) of foods you might like to try in the Ingredient Inspiration section - it's helpful for giving you new ideas for seasonal produce, or if you're craving something in particular.

I've tried to strike a balance between giving alternative measurements, without cluttering up the text. I am a classic confused UK cook – I weigh myself in pounds, measure myself in feet and inches, but cook in grams, especially since 5:2 because the measurements seem more precise. I apologise in advance for any inconsistencies.

160

There are lots of conversion sites on the internet but I find this one (bit.ly/U6n2hV) the simplest and least cluttered for metric to imperial – and this page converts grams to US cups (bit.ly/U4Ft6A).

Food and Fasting Tips

Measure, measure, measure (at least till you get used to it!)

Yes, it's a bit tedious but it can also be very enlightening - see more on how to measure in Part Two. It will really give you an insight into why we might be consuming more calories than we ever realised before. Weighing and then recording *exactly* what you're eating on the Fast Days – right down to a teaspoon of balsamic vinegar or a sprinkling of sunflower seeds – is the best way to avoid the temptation to cheat. Of course, once you're more used to the quantities you can eat on Fast Days, you won't need to measure so frequently.

Doll's House meals

The simplest way to do this diet is cut out all snacks, and then measure out and eat the tiniest portions of the foods you and your family normally eat. Use smaller plates or dishes - I think of my Fast Day yogurt and fruit as a doll's house-sized portion. Sometimes it's easier than cooking something entirely separate.

Vitamin 'Insurance'

It makes sense to take a multi-vitamin during the fasts, just to make sure you're getting enough nutrients. Of course, if you're eating lots of vegetables, you might be getting even higher levels of certain vitamins than usual, but I think taking a good multi-vitamin is a sensible move for anyone who is dieting.

Meal replacement shakes and bars

There's no need to buy 'special' foods for your Fast Days, and personally I prefer to eat foods that are similar to what I eat on normal days - just smaller portions or with fewer 'naughty' additions.

Having said this, diet shakes, soups and bars have proved useful for some people - they are fortified with vitamins, and they also offer very precise calorie-controlled portions, so you know exactly what you're getting. They're recommended by James Johnson for his Alternate Day Diet because they're easy but also because they're so boring – he thinks they reduce the inclination to eat. For me, they'd reduce the inclination to do the diet at all but others have found it useful to go that way.

So if you enjoy them or find them convenient, there's no reason why you shouldn't use them - so long as you eat normally the rest of the time!

Savouring the flavour

Unless you have chosen meal replacements, one good way to make your Fast Days more enjoyable is finding ways to add flavour without adding too many calories: which means that spices, fresh herbs, and lower-calorie sauces come into their own to add depth and keep your taste buds entertained. Take your pick from:

Chilli - flakes are brilliant for pepping up soups, stews and baked beans – one study also suggests they might help with fat-burning and increasing the metabolism (bit.ly/11jyZHs). But go easy - they pack a punch. Fresh chillies are delicious too but need even more caution.

Hot Chilli Sauce - is another easy way to liven things up. It contains more calories than the flakes but you need very little.

Horseradish/Wasabi - I love the scary-hot tang of wasabi (the green horseradish you get in pre-packed sushi or in a tube) even though the tiniest quantity is eye-watering. Great to take your mind off fasting, though!

Mustard - like horseradish, it's hot and tasty and works with cheese, ham and other cold meats.

Fresh Herbs - great as an addition to a salad: the most versatile are chives and basil. Try chives with scrambled eggs or with other herbs in an omelette, basil torn up and added to tomato-based soups or stews/sauces, and rocket or young spinach leaf works well both as a salad crop and added to soup or stews to add body and taste.

Soy sauce - is salty but definitely adds zing, as does Worcestershire sauce (which is not strictly vegetarian, due to the anchovies - but you can get a veggie version if it bothers you).

Vinegars - cider or wine vinegars can work well as a dressing without oil, as can balsamic, though the latter is slightly more calorific as it's sweet, so measure it and count in your calorie allowance - it's around 16 cals per tablespoon. I also love tomatoes baked in the oven with a few drops of balsamic and then served with herbs.

Garlic - low in calories and a little goes a very long way. It's much less potent if you roast it along with other vegetables - break into cloves but leave them in their pink skins till they're roasted, then use as a puree. You can even spread on a slice of bread if you're brave, it's as unctuous as butter.

Miso - this Japanese fermented paste comes in jars or tubes and adds a meaty (though it's veggie) flavour to all sorts of dishes, and also works as a very low calorie soup stirred with boiling water in a mug. You can also buy it as powdered sachets ready to make into soup - more convenient to take to work.

Salsas - either buy fresh, in jars (still surprisingly tasty) or make your own (see the recipe under Ingredient Inspiration) - it's great as an accompaniment to fish, lean meat or Quorn/Veggie burgers and as it contains no sugar, is a much better bet than tomato ketchup.

Pickles/chutneys - I am addicted to all things sweet and sour, including pickles and chutneys. Be mindful of the sugar content, but a small amount, calorie-counted, can give you a hit of flavour - spread some very thinly on a slice of bread, add a slice of low-cal cheese and grill for a Fast Day cheese on toast...

What NOT to eat on your Fast Day

Of course, you can eat what you like - up to your calorie limit - but here are some things that many people avoid on Fast Days:

Fruit and Fruit Juice

Juiced and many whole fruits may upset your blood sugar balance due to the natural sugars - you could be hit by cravings by 11am which is NOT what you want. The main exception would be berries - strawberries, blueberries and raspberries won't give you quite the same intense sugar hit, but they are intensely flavoured. Frozen berries can also work well - blueberries and raspberries are particularly nice.

Refined Carbohydrates

White bread, potatoes and white rice are particularly likely to give you that carb high that will then make you hungry 'on the rebound'. Complex carbohydrates - seeded rolls, brown rice, sweet potatoes - will have a less dramatic effect but you won't get a very big portion of these foods if you want to stay within your Fast Day calorie limit. And not everyone feels the same - one dieter swears by a small jacket potato as her main meal.

If you're interested in reading more, you can read more at bit.ly/Tv2B2Y about how a food's Glycaemic Index (the rate at which sugar is released to the blood) can affect cravings and hunger pangs.

Alcoholic Drinks

These are high in calories and won't fill you up - on an empty stomach, they could lower your willpower, too.

Confession time: I know it's nothing to be proud of, but I have been known to save 100 cals for a decent glass of wine if I am going to the pub. Obviously, you shouldn't be having 20% of your calories as alcohol on a regular basis but wine or particularly brut champagne/cava can be a very nice pick-me-up. Two glasses, though, and you probably won't be able to resists what everyone else is eating...

Breakfasts

For years, received diet wisdom has been that breakfast is the most important meal of the day – but I'm one of many 5:2 dieters to discover that I don't actually need it.

However, if you can't face the day without it (and in the 'Horizon' programme, Dr Mosley eats Breakfast and Dinner), there are lots of options for you.

Ready-Made Options

With ready-made breakfast options, it makes sense to get label-savvy – so many cereals are high in sugar that they could really knock you off course.

Cereals

Many 5:2 dieters avoid sweetened packet cereals, due to the blood sugar high/low that I mentioned in the introduction to this part of the book. Also the portions when you measure them out are really tiny. Porridge or All Bran are probably a better bet, or some low-sugar mueslis including mainstream brands like Alpen – there are some great guidelines to how to analyse ingredients to find a lower GI cereal here at bit.ly/QPcolf_

Cereal bars

These are marketed as healthy alternatives to normal

cereals, but have many of the same drawbacks – most come in at 100 calories or so but are so sweet you'll be craving another one within an hour or less. A test of cereal bars carried out by *Which* in the UK showed that one contained almost 4 teaspoons' worth of sugar.

Porridge/Oatmeal

Nutritionists often recommend oats as a good breakfast cereal because they release energy in the body slowly. For portion control, a pre-measured packet like Oatso Simple or Quaker Instant Oatmeal works well for some dieters. It's better to make it with water to save calories, but if you can't bear it, semi-skimmed milk will still keep the calories under 200.

Oatso Simple Original with water

98 calories

Oatso Simple Original with 180mg semi-skimmed milk

188 calories

Quaker Instant Oatmeal, Lower Sugar Flavours

120 calories

Quaker Oatmeal Perfect Portions Cinnamon Instant Oatmeal

160 calories

Out and about, Pret a Manger do a **Porridge with Compote** for 267 calories or without for 242 calories - a hefty chunk out of your allowance, but filling and easy. **Starbucks Perfect Porridge with Skimmed Milk** is 205 for a pot, as **is Sainsbury's Express Porridge Pot. In the US, Starbucks Perfect Oatmeal is 140 calories without all the extras – I'd definitely advise against the brown sugar. The McDonald's oatmeal is pretty high in calories at 270 for the Apple and Cinnamon variety.** See below for home-made versions.

Smoothies

Pure fruit smoothies might seem tempting for a meal on the go, but they are not ideal, for the reasons given in the previous chapter – fruit can play havoc with blood sugar and make you hungry very fast. But those with yogurt, oats and other slowly-digested ingredients may be a better bet. Look at the calorie counts but also at the sugar/carbohydrate count on the label - the lower the better.

Yogurt

There are so many varieties of yogurt that it's impossible to generalise on whether it's a good option. The label will be a clue, but it's often a good option to buy a natural low-fat, low-carb yogurt and then add a few nuts or seeds (again, measured carefully) to stave off hunger pangs later: sunflower or pumpkin seeds will work, along with a few fresh strawberries or raspberries in season.

Home-Made and Home-Cooked

Something on Toast...

Who can resist toast...? It's the crack cocaine of the carbohydrate world for me, so it can be a risky choice on a fast day. But if you can stick to one or two slices without butter it can make your mornings more bearable. A medium slice of Hovis Granary Wholemeal is 92 cals: a slice from one of their smaller wholemeal loaves is around 57 . In the US, a slice of Wonder Cottage White is 80 calories and Wonder Stoneground is 90.

The following are for the topping only and I've used a range of different brands - most supermarkets will have similar products:

Food	Calories
Medium poached egg	75-85
Heinz Snap Pot Baked Beans 200g	144
Heinz - Home Style Beans (Chipotle BBQ Style) ½ cup	130
Sunpat Crunchy Peanut Butter - 1 teaspoon	30

Food	Calories
(5g)	
Skippy Natural Creamy Peanut Butter	31
Philadelphia - 1/3 Less Fat (Than Cream Cheese) Chive & Onion 1 tablespoon (15g)	35
Philadelphia Extra Light Cream Cheese (10g)	11
Philadelphia with Cadbury Dairy Milk (10g)	30
Deli sliced boiled ham	80
Tesco - Sliced Honey Roast Ham	24
Kraft Singles American Cheese Slices	60
Tesco Reduced Flat Cheese Slice (25g)	75

<u>Go to work on an egg?</u>

Eggs are protein-rich, but they can also be very satisfying, especially at breakfast, so it's worth considering them. Poaching or boiling are the least calorific ways of preparing them, but they can also be fried using the oil sprays you can buy, which typically work out at 1 calorie per spray - not as tasty as butter, but they won't eat up your entire allowance either.

Basic scrambled egg recipe: 155 calories

Take two eggs (1 50g/US large egg has approx. 70 calories), crack into a mug or cup, add 2 tablespoons (30ml : 15 calories) of semi-skimmed milk.

Beat well with a fork till yolks and whites are combined. Season with salt and pepper.

Spray a small non-stick saucepan with low-calorie or no-calorie spray and put on low/medium heat: the more slowly you cook them, the less rubbery they'll be.

Add egg mixture and cook for one minute without beating. Then begin to move the mix around the pan with a spoon or spatula, until mixture begins to set or thicken, depending on how you prefer your eggs. Cook thoroughly if you are pregnant or immune-compromised. Remember mixture will keep heating as long as it's in the hot pan so serve immediately.

Additions:

- Fresh herbs, chopped
- Chilli flakes
- Mushrooms pre-fried in no-cal spray
- Chopped ham or smoked salmon – a little goes a long way

Serving suggestion: Instead of serving on toast, use no-cal spray to fry large Portobello/field mushrooms for 4-5 minutes (turning halfway) - and top with the eggs.

Omelettes are great, too, partly because to me they seem more complete without the addition of the (calorific) toast.

Basic Omelette recipe: 140 calories

Break two medium/50g eggs (70 cals) into a bowl and whisk well till combined. Season with salt and pepper.

Use a small non-stick frying or omelette pan and no/low-cal spray and heat the pan till it's hot but not burning: apparently you should be able to touch it with the back of your hand but I would caution against doing this!!!

Add the egg and keep the mix moving so that all the uncooked egg has contact with the pan – do this for 1-2 minutes.

Then hold the pan at an angle and let the omelette move forwards towards the site of the pan – use the spatula to lift a third of the omelette back on itself. It's a folding process! Do it again for the other side until it's a cigar shape!

Again, you can add extras, either to the centre of the omelette when it's part cooked but before the fold, or to the basic mixture.

Home-made Porridge/Oatmeal

There are many different brands available, so pick your favourite: I am a huge fan of Flavahan's Irish Porridge Oats - they are so creamy and yummy, even made with water.

Oatmeal brands have microwave or hob cooking instructions on the pack. A 40g serving of Flavahan's made with 240nl skimmed milk is 237 calories.

Things to add to porridge/oatmeal

Food	Calories
Teaspoon honey	20
Teaspoon (5g) sunflower seeds	30
Teaspoon (5g) dried sultanas	15
½ grated very small apple (approx. 50g)	27
Raspberries - 20 (frozen are fine: add them to unheated oats straight from the freezer before cooking when fresh berries aren't available)	20 (1 cal each!)
Blueberries: 50 berries	39
Tablespoon (15g) low-fat yogurt	Check label!
Cadbury Bournville Cocoa powder 1 teaspoon	18
Teaspoon of powdered cinnamon (a teaspoon may be too much!)	6

Home-made Bircher Muesli

This is how I like my oats. I first discovered it on holiday in the posh hotel buffet, and it's filling and healthy. It's also almost effortless and tastes a lot yummier than it sounds. The only problem is that it makes a very small portion in a bowl... but we're getting used to those doll's house-sized portions.

Basic Bircher Muesli: 168 calories

This is a small portion but very filling...

25g porridge oats (97 cals)
25ml semi skimmed milk (12 cals) or apple juice
(11cals) plus a teaspoon (5g) of sultanas (15cals)
Mix the two together, put in a bowl or plastic container in the fridge overnight, covered.
In the morning, if it's a little bit dry, add slightly more liquid. Grate half a small apple over the top (27 cals), mix in and 2 tablespoons (30ml) of plain low-fat yogurt (17 cals) plus any of the ingredients suggested above for porridge - berries are especially good).
Take it to work in a plastic pot!

Cool Lunches and Hot Dinners

Again, I've split this into ready-made meals that I and other dieters have found filling and tasty - and then suggestions for home-made dishes. You can obviously have them for lunch, dinner - or breakfast, if you feel like it. It's your diet...

Ready Made

Main dishes

If you choose to eat one main meal a day, then it will be really easy to find ready meals that come in at 500-600 calories a serving. As a pointer, try to choose menus with a balance of protein and carbohydrate, to keep you from getting hungry again too quickly (a chocolate cheesecake or brownie dessert might come in under the limit but will probably drive you crazy with hunger again within a couple of hours).

If you're veering towards eating two or three meals a day, here are some of the dishes dieters have recommended. Do be careful though – labels can be deceptive, as Kirsty discovered:

> *If it looks too good to be true it probably is.*
> *I picked up a ready meal where the label*
> *said 440 calories – but when I looked*

closer, that was per serving, i.e. for half of it!! That'll be tea tomorrow then.

UK Options

Innocent Veg Pots - you'll either love or loathe these vegetable and pulse-based dishes, which tend to be stews or casseroles based on various cuisines, including Indian, Thai and Mexican. They are packed with veg and can be quite filling, though the presence of lots of beans and fibre can have explosive consequences... just saying. The calorie count varies from around 215 to over 300. Many supermarkets now do own brand versions.

Kirstys.co.uk - get the thumbs up from several 5:2 regulars: these healthy versions of classic dishes come from the company featured on TV's 'Dragon's Den'. They're stocked in UK supermarkets (Sainsbury's at the time of writing) and particular favourites are... Moroccan Vegetables with Quinoa (276 calories) and Cottage Pie with Sweet Potato Mash (288 calories)

Marks & Spencer Simply Fuller Longer range does what it says on the packet, and the dishes are formulated to satisfy the appetite for as long as possible. They're not all low-calorie so do check the label – the fish dishes tend to be the lowest in calories e.g. King Prawns, Lochmuir Hot Smoked Salmon With Couscous & A Lemon Vinaigrette is 320 calories!

> **Waitrose's Love Life You Count** range has its fans: they do apply the branding to a lot of different products but the You Count ones tend to offer a main meal dish at less than 300 calories.

Most supermarkets make vegetable-based side dishes which come in smaller packs than the standard ready meals. They're often designed for sharing, but eating the whole pack of Cauliflower Cheese or one of the Indian side dishes can still come in at under 300 cals and often the dishes are satisfying in themselves. I like the Spinach Dhal from Waitrose - the spices in veggie side dishes mean your meal is big on flavour, but low in calories.

One tip: If you choose a diet option ready-meal, try adding your own spices or fresh herbs to add flavour - I've mixed in a little French or wholegrain mustard into a thin cauliflower cheese sauce which had no discernible cheese, or you could add just a little low-fat cream cheese to a sauce or curry side dish without adding too many calories... soy or chilli sauces are also great.

US Options

The ready-meals market is smaller in the US, but the following frozen dishes are lower in calories than traditional versions of the same dishes: do read the labels for salt and other additives.

The Lean Cuisine (leancuisine.com) range has a vast set of choices, including the 'spa collection' and over ninety without preservatives, including Grilled Chicken Primavera at 220 calories or Hunan Stir-Fry with Beef at 280 cals. Read the reviews to find out which dieters enjoy!

Smart Ones from Weight Watchers (eatyourbest.com) includes a Satisfying Selections Range which is designed to keep you full with extra protein: it includes Peppercorn Beef at 280 calories. There's also a star rating system on the website so you can see what other people have liked – the Chicken in Spicy Peanut Sauce gets a high rating, and is 250 cals.

The Healthy Choice (healthychoice.com) range includes a vegetarian range, free of additives, with dishes like Pumpkin Squash Ravioli at 310 calories. The Cafe Steamers get the thumbs up especially the Honey Glazed Turkey and Sweet Potatoes at 250 calories. Lots of reviews on this site, too.

Kashi Frozen meals (kashi.com) are less widely available but have an emphasis on whole grains, like Sesame Chicken and Pilaf at 300 calories, and Amy's Kitchen (amys.com) also has its fans, with lots of vegetarian and gluten-free options. The cheese enchilada is gluten free and has 240 calories.

Soups

Making your own soup is easy and cheap, but for a no-hassle option, I often buy ready-made and the flavours and brands keep on improving (they used to taste very salty but I find the newer versions less heavy handed). It's a great option in colder weather when a salad, however low in calories, doesn't quite seem to fill you up. There's evidence at bbc.in/YahY4T_ that supports the experience many people have of feeling full up for longer after soup, too.

UK Options

One brand that gets the thumbs up is the **Glorious Skinny** - the Azteca is spicy, with chunks of pepper and tortilla (half a pot = 90 cals), while the Fragrant Thai Carrot is very warming and 119 calories for a portion.

The Yorkshire Provender Company has some lovely dishes. Pepper and Wensleydale is a little higher in calories than some (201 calories for half a pot), but the chewy pieces of cheese are delicious. Beetroot and Horseradish comes in at 168 cals for half a pot.

Supermarket own brand soups - still in the plastic tubs which you can microwave - tend to be a little bit cheaper I like the **Marks & Spencer** Spicy Red Lentil and Tomato which is 150 cals. for half a pot, but incredibly filling.

Don't rule out Cup-a-soups or tinned soups – your

favourites will still most likely be really low in calories compared to other options!

I often eat a portion of soup for lunch and dinner - with a slice of bread or Ryvita to add some crunch (I noticed when I tried to eat only soup, I missed the texture of other foods as much as the calories). Again, I like the convenience of having my day's meals in a single pot - great for work.

US Options

Again, the fresh soups market doesn't exist in the same way in the US, but there are still plenty of options.

The Wal-Mart Marketside range includes a number of 'fresh' soup options without additives in microwaveable containers. It includes a Vegetable Soup at 90 calories per serving, and Chicken Vegetable Pasta at 100 per serving. Campbell's (campbellsoup.com) have an extensive selection of soups, including a Healthy Request range with dishes like Mexican-Style Chicken Tortilla Soup at 110 calories per portion, and many of them are available in microwave packs to take to work.

There's also the GO range which has chunkier soups served in pouches, like the Spicy Chorizo & Pulled Chicken with Black Beans at 210 cals for the pack.

Grains and Noodles

Pasta won't offer you much bulk for your calories, but if you want something more solid than soup, and as convenient, you could look at the microwaveable rice pouches which have extra flavours and spicing built in - one of these will probably add up to around 400 cals for the packet, so serve in two portions, perhaps with some frozen veg added: I'd definitely gravitate towards the brown rice versions as white rice will usually make you hungry again, much faster.

In the UK, Tilda Roasted Pepper and Courgette Steamed Brown Basmati Rice contains 176 calories for half a pack, or the Veetee Vegetable Biryani is 174 for half a pack. In the US, there's Uncle Ben's Spanish Style, for example, at 200 calories for half a pack.

We're moving towards Home-Made in this category but there's been a lot of talk on diet forums lately about 'no calorie' shirataki noodles which are made of a kind of yam and are supposed to leave you full but not add to your calorie count. They're so popular they've been sold out wherever I go but I've heard mixed reports. Yes, they're filling, and they can work well combined with a stir fry or some prawns or lean meat. However, don't expect them to taste too much like 'real' noodles. They can also have a slightly fishy smell. Shirataki noodles are also available with tofu as part of the mix which may make them more satisfying. You can buy them online or via health food or Asian speciality shops.

Preparing couscous could count as borderline cooking, but there are various flavoured couscous brands that you put in a bowl and add boiling water to – in the UK, the Ainsley Harriott packets contain two portions of around 170-190 each - again, you can bulk them out with frozen peas or corn, or serve with a veggie sausage or burger.

Home-Made and Home-Cooked

All the egg dishes and 'on toast' dishes from the Breakfast Section will work equally well at another time of day: beans on toast is one of those dishes you can eat without anyone really noticing you're on a diet - especially nice if you add some chilli flakes or sauce!

The best site I've found to allow you to select favourite ingredients, cooking time and calorie counts is the BBC Good Food site, bbcgoodfood.com – there's a specific section with recommended 200-400 calorie dishes via bit.ly/SsvbkI including Healthy Fish and Chips, and Full English Frittata. You can also save all your favourites into your own recipe binder if you register, and read other reviews of each recipe posted by users.

In this section, I'll stick to simple dishes which barely count as 'recipes' – they're more suggestions for fast and easy meals when you don't want to spend too much time cooking or in reach of temptations.

Meat and Two Veg

You obviously need to be a little more careful about your meat and two veg meals while you're fasting, but it certainly doesn't mean giving them up!

Here are some suggestions for combinations and portion size: treat all the calorie counts as a guideline and double check on the back of your packs. Most steamed/boiled green veg come in at around 30-35 calories per 100 grams though peas and corn are higher in calories.

Meat/Fish	Veg 1	Veg 2	Total cals:
Salmon Portion size: small steak, 100g, **135 calories**	Mange tout/ snow peas 100g – 32 calories	Mushrooms fried in no-cal spray 60g 10 calories	177
Tuna Portion size: 1 steak, 75g: **115 calories**	Sweet corn 75g canned 50 cals	Spinach ½ cup cooked & drained 32 cals	197
Prawns Portion size: 100g, **80 calories**	Roast tomatoes 10 cherry tomatoes 30 cals roasted with no cal spray & 5ml balsamic 5 cals	Green beans 100g approx. 30 cals	145

Chicken Portion size: 100g breast fillet, **100-140 calories**	Broccoli 1 cup, steamed 30 cals	Sliced mixed peppers 80g 25 cals	155-195
Turkey Portion size: 100g breast fillet, **100-140 calories**	Baby Carrots Frozen handful 80g 18 cals	Cauliflower 100g steamed 25 cals	143-183
Quorn burger/banger: Portion size: Burger 50g, **80 calories** banger x 1 **50-60 calories**	Sweet potato (small: 133g) 105 calories	Garden peas 50 34 cals	189-219

One Pot/Pan/Dish meals

The recipes that follow are simple and fresh and infinitely adaptable: use them as the basis for healthy, nutritious and low-calorie meals on Fast Days.

Easy Vegetable Curry 150 calories per portion (makes two portions)

Replace the veg with any others in season – adjusting the calories, of course. Also, you can serve with a portion of meat or fish as listed in the previous section.

> 1 teaspoon (5ml) oil
>
> 2 cloves garlic, crushed
>
> 1 onion, finely chopped
>
> 1tsp Chilli Powder
>
> 1tsp Ground Ginger
>
> 1tsp Turmeric Powder
>
> 100g Green Beans, sliced
>
> 200g Cauliflower or Broccoli, broken into small florets
>
> 100g Carrots, sliced
>
> 100g Potatoes, diced
>
> 1tsp Tomato Puree
>
> 20g Sultanas

Cook the garlic and onion in the oil in a large pan for five minutes, before adding the spices and cooking gently for a further minute. Add all the vegetables and 300ml of water, then add the other ingredients. Heat till water boils, then reduce the heat and cover – it'll be ready in half an hour. It keeps well in the fridge for forty-eight hours if you want to save till your next Fast Day.

Mediterranean Roast Veg: 148 calories per portion (makes four portions)

This is good with whatever herbs or spices you fancy – try chilli flakes. Mushrooms, baby corn or slices of butternut squash (in 1 cm slices so they bake through) taste great too. If you make more than you need, make soup: add to a large saucepan with water and a tin of tomatoes, bring to the boil. Adjust the water to make the consistency you like. When it's cooled down, blend in pan with a stick blender.

> 3 tbsp. olive oil
>
> 4 large courgettes sliced
>
> 5 plum tomatoes sliced
>
> 2 aubergines sliced
>
> 1 large garlic bulb (don't peel)
>
> A bunch of rosemary, broken into sprigs, or oregano, or thyme

Heat oven to 220C/200C fan/gas 7. Drizzle a third of the oil into a tin or ovenproof dish then layer the vegetables across the dish – with the garlic head in the middle. Poke the herbs in amongst the layered veg, add 1 tablespoon of olive oil over the top and season.

Roast for 45 minutes – 1 hour until the vegetables are charred around the edges, adding remaining oil during cooking. You can use less but it's virtuous already!
Serve with the still-wrapped cloves of garlic, to be squeezed out over the vegetables.

So Easy Stir Fry: 160 calories per portion (makes 2 very generous portions)

Another base recipe that you can adapt with different veg – peppers and spring onion/scallion would be nice. Or buy stir-fry veg packs from supermarkets/convenience stores. If you want to use meat or fish, pre-fry these in the oil to make sure they're cooked through. Then set aside, fry veg in the same pan and heat through all the ingredients after adding soy and chilli sauce. Alternatively, add thinly sliced tofu with the vegetables, or a beaten egg, just after the soy and chilli sauce stage for veggie protein options.

> 1 tbsp. vegetable oil
>
> 1 red chilli, sliced (leave out if you don't like hot food)
>
> 1 garlic clove, sliced
>
> 500g mixed vegetables such as pak choi, baby corn and broccoli
>
> 1½ tbsp. soy sauce
>
> 2 tbsp. sweet chilli sauce

Heat the oil in a wok or frying pan, then fry the chilli and garlic for one min. Add the vegetables and make sure they've all been coated in all. Fry for 2-3 mins, then add the soy and chilli sauce then cook for a further 2-3 mins until the veg are tender.

Soups

Spicy Indian Lentil & Tomato: 130 calories per portion (makes 2 portions)

A very simple, warming soup made from the things you have in your larder. Double up the portions and freeze if you like.

> 1 chopped onion
> Pinch of chilli flakes
> 2 tablespoons of red lentils
> 1 400g tin chopped tomatoes
> 500ml vegetable stock (I used Marigold bouillon)
> Coriander/cilantro leaf, to taste (maybe ½ bunch)

Put all the ingredients, except the coriander, in a pan together and heat till simmering. Cover and cook for twenty minutes till the lentils are soft, then add the coriander/cilantro, cook for one minute and blend with stick blender. Season and serve.

Mushroom tom yum soup: 40 calories per portion (makes 4 portions)

Very tasty, very fast and very low in calories.

1 litre chicken or vegetable stock

1-2 tbsp. tom yum paste

200g fresh mushrooms (ideally a mixture including oyster and shiitake)

4 dried shiitake mushrooms rehydrated in water (remove hard edges)

Juice of 1 lime

Fish sauce to taste – around 1 tablespoon

1 sliced red chilli

Coriander/cilantro to taste

Bring the stock to the boil in a large pan, add the paste and then the mushrooms. Simmer for five minutes before adding the other ingredients. Season and add more fish sauce if required before serving.

Green and White Super Soup: 76 calories per portion (makes 2 portions)

Super-vitamins, super-easy.

½ bunch spring onions, chopped

1 teaspoon oil

1 small potato, peeled and diced

500ml vegetable stock (made with 5g Marigold bouillon)

140g bag watercress, spinach and rocket

Cook the spring onions/scallions in olive oil until soft: add the potato and cook for two more minutes, then add stock and simmer till potato is tender (10-15 minutes depending on size of the dice). Add the bag of salad, simmer for a minute then use stick blender to blend till smooth. Season and serve.

Almost Instant Corn Chowder: 115 calories per portion (1 portion)

1 medium spring onion/scallion

300 ml stock made with 2.5g/ ½ teaspoon Marigold Swiss Vegetable Bouillon

100g frozen sweet corn

Pinch chilli flakes

Fresh semi-skimmed/2% fat milk

Use no-cal spray to fry the onion. Add all the ingredients except the milk, simmer for five minutes, then add milk and blend lightly with stick blender. Season & serve.

Stuffed vegetables

Vegetables make ideal 'carriers' for ingredients – low in calories but colourful and tasty for Fast Days!

Portabello/breakfast mushrooms are large and flat, as big as beef burgers, and make brilliant containers for fillings. I tend to grill or microwave them with the fillings – they're so low in calories that you could also serve them as 'burgers' if they've been grilled or fried in no-cal spray, in a bun!

Philly Mushrooms: 66 calories for 2

Take 2 large flat mushrooms (approx. 125g: 20 calories) and wipe with kitchen towel. Spoon 30g (2tbsp) Philadelphia Light with Herbs or Chives into the mushrooms and top with chopped herbs or black pepper: either grill for 2 minutes until hot through or microwave for 30-45 seconds.

The Mediterranean filling for the avocado recipe below also works well in mushrooms or peppers.

Stuffed Avocado: 125 plus your choice of filling

Avocados are high in fat but filling and tasty – you can serve them cold, of course, but also hot if you want to try something different. Their shape makes a nice 'bowl' for all sorts of fillings. Use half a medium Hass avocado (125 calories: save the other half in the fridge to use later the same day - store with the stone still inside and a little lemon juice on the cut surface to stop it discolouring) and add whatever fillings you fancy:

- Guacamole style: add shop-bought salsa, or a mix of two cherry chopped tomatoes, sprinkling of chilli flakes, and half a chopped medium spring onion (less than 10 calories)
- Cream cheese style: add 1 tablespoon of Philadelphia light (any flavour, 20 calories) – this can be microwaved for approx. 20-30 seconds or grilled for approx. 5 minutes to serve as a kind of pate with Ryvita or other crackers: spray first with 0-cal cooking spray before grilling.
- Rocket and balsamic vinegar: pour 1tbsp (15ml: 15 cals) vinegar into the hollow of the avocado, add a good handful of rocket leaves (20g is loads and just 4 cals) and grind plenty of pepper and sea salt on top.
- Prawns and lime: 60g of cooked prawns (approx. 45 cals) plus half a lime (under 10 cals for the juice) to serve. Or use low-cal dressing of your choice.
- Mediterranean Hot: spray the avocado with no-cal cooking spray and grill for five minutes or microwave for 20-30 seconds. In the hollow, place

a mix of 1 chopped sun-dried tomato with oil drained off, two stoned olives, a few capers, ½ spring onion/scallion, some torn basil or rocket leaves (filling is less than 20 calories).

Quickest ever stuffed pepper: 92 for two halves

Halve a medium red or yellow pepper (31 calories) and pull out seeds/ white core. Add three cherry tomatoes to each half (18 calories for 6) and medium spring onion/scallion, (5 cals) cut into small slices with a knife or scissors. Top with 30g Philadelphia Light (any savoury flavour, 40 calories) plus other flavourings from suggested in the Tips section.

Grill for approx. 10-12 minutes or roast in oven 200c for around 30 minutes, till the pepper flesh is soft and the edges are charred.

Salads

A pre-washed bag of salad contains very few calories – and is a canvas for a great Fast Day salad.

Salad Ingredient	Calories
½ bag pre-washed salad – whichever you like!	15-30: see label
Cherry tomatoes	3 per tomato
Sliced bell pepper	30 per pepper
Beetroot, 50g cooked	16
Sweet corn – 50g drained from tin	40-50
Spring onion / scallion	Medium – 8
Parmesan – great shaved thinly with potato slicer	10g shavings 40
Cottage cheese: varies depending on fat content	60-100 per 100g
Wafer thin ham (deli style) – slice varies	10-15 per slice
Wafer thin turkey (deli style) – slice varies	8-15 per slice
Cooked prawns	50g = 40
Smoked salmon – 1 60g slice	80-100
Artichoke hearts: depends on size of can	25-50 per portion
Pumpkin seeds: teaspoon (5g)	29
Pine nuts: teaspoon (5g)	35
Sunflower seeds: teaspoon (5g)	30
Buffalo mozzarella, ½ container (2.2 oz/60g.)	170
Chopped apple: ½ small apple (approx. 50g)	27
Walnuts: teaspoon (5g)	34
Whole boiled egg	70-80

A-Z Ingredient Inspiration

This section is designed to give you a little boost if you're bored and are looking for quick, new ideas.

Food	Ideas	Calories
A is for Asparagus	Super nutritious and filling, and delicious, either steamed, boiled or - easiest of all - microwaved. Serve with sea salt and pepper, lemon juice, or a nice poached egg on the side to dip into! You can also pre-cook and then grill. It's a great summer dish.	5 spears = 25
A is also for Almonds	These are *so* good and although like all nuts they're calorific, a small handful can be very filling. I've also used them ground – a teaspoon mixed with yogurt and berries, gives you a hint of sweetness while containing negligible carbs, so you'll stave off the hunger pangs for longer.	1 whole = 7 1 Teaspoon = (5g) 31
B is for Beetroot	You might have gathered that I am a bit of a beetroot fiend, especially the sort that's been flavoured with chilli, or baked with cumin powder and served with a little low-fat yogurt or cumin. It's very good for you, and makes a delicious salad with rocket,	50g cooked = 16

	cherry tomatoes, balsamic vinegar and some chopped fresh apple. I also like it with fresh mozzarella - the kind that comes floating in water.	
B is also for Broccoli	Another one of those super-foods. Horrible over-cooked, but steaming works well, or have you tried frying till it almost goes black? The edges caramelise if you slice through the florets into 3mm/1/4 inch slices, then heat some spray oil in a pan till very hot, and fry on both sides. You need the extractor fan for this one or an open window as it can smoke but it's great with pepper and sea salt, soy sauce or chilli sauce, and very low in calories.	100g= 38
C is for Chocolate	Yum. Etc. You can't have too much of it, but two or four squares of the dark, expensive kind can be enough to satisfy a craving. It's sweet, but not too sweet, and high in anti-oxidants, too.	10g (4 small squares) = 58
D is for Dijon mustard	Or any kind of mustard. I add it to lots of savoury dishes to give a low-calorie kick - there are calories in it but it's so hot that you only need a little.	1 teaspoon (5ml) = 15

E is for Edamame beans	Those whole pods that are served in Asian restaurants are available frozen to eat at home, and they're filling, nutritious and can satisfy a snack craving.	50g = 61
F is for low-fat Feta cheese	This has a strong, salty taste, so a little goes a long way. Try in a Greek salad with lots of tomato, black olives and cucumber, perhaps with some red wine vinegar or a ready-made lower calorie dressing.	50g = 100-120
G is for Ginger	One of your best friends for extra flavour during Fast Days. I am a big fan of the clean taste of pickled ginger that's served with sushi – I'm addicted to it on its own!	25g (plenty!) = `10-15
H is for Ham	Great for when you're having a savoury craving. Parma is posh, try 2 slices of Parma ham with 6 thin slices of melon.	For melon and ham = 80
I is for Ices	They don't have to be out of bounds if you choose carefully. A Solero is the dieter's friend on hot days or look for Italian style ice-cream (typically less fatty than American style) or a	Solero = 90 1 2.5 oz. scoop Baskin Robbins Fat

	creamy low-fat frozen yogurt (check the calories though as some can be higher than normal ice-cream).	Free Vanilla Frozen Yogurt = 80
J is for Jelly	Sugar-free jellies can help overcome a sweet craving with negligible calories.	3-10
K is for Kiwi Fruits	Often overlooked - maybe because of their unpromising exterior. But inside there's a frenzy of vitamin C.	46
L is for Lentils	Cheap red lentils make a great basis for soup – see the recipe - and the 'gourmet' Puy variety are extremely filling and provide a nutritious and tasty base for a salad.	100g ready to eat Puy lentils = 130
M is for Marmite	Definitely one for the Brits here – we all know that a little of this yeasty spread goes a long way. Great on crisp breads or a single slice of toast. I also like Marmite flavoured cheese bites too: 85 calories for a portion.	10 for a 4g spread
N is for Noodles	Try the Shirataki 'no calorie' noodles which can be found in the chiller section and contain fewer than 20 cals (sometimes none at all) per serving. The ones with tofu taste less 'fishy' and it's best to use a strong flavoured	Less than 20 cals per serving

	sauce and also to 'dry roast' them for a minute in a hot pan before using!	
O is for Oreo Cookies	Maybe it's because they look so cute but I adore Oreos – and the mini biscuits can give you a sweet hit without too many calories if you can stop at one or two	½ 29g Bite size pack (4 cookies) = 65
P is for Popsicles	Make your own low-cal popsicles or ice lollies with sugar-free squash, diluted fruit juice, low-fat yogurt or pureed fruit. Use a reusable mould and go wild!	Depends on what you add
Q is for Quinoa	Quinoa – which those in the know pronounce 'keen-wa' is a seed originally grown by the Incas which is used as a grain in pilaffs or as a stuffing. It's very high protein so a little will fill you up and you can use it in salads or other dishes that are normally made with rice.	100g cooked = 100-110
R is for Ricotta	A lovely light Italian cheese with a mousse-like texture for dips, sauces or even as a substitute for mayonnaise in salads which need 'binding.' Check labels to get lower calorie versions.	1 cup = 50-100 depending on brand

S is for Salsa	The shop bought stuff can be really good but nothing beats home-made: this one improves after a day in the fridge. 1 tomato, finely diced 1 medium red (bell) pepper ½ cucumber, & ½ celery stick, finely diced 1 medium onion, chopped finely 2 tablespoons vinegar 2 tablespoons salt Pinch each chilli flakes, black pepper, oregano 1 teaspoon Worcestershire sauce Soak the onions in the vinegar and 1 tablespoon of salt. Leave overnight. Roast the bell pepper till the skin is charred, discard seeds and white parts, chop and add to the other chopped vegetables and onions. Add flavourings. Makes 8 portions.	14 cals per portion
T is for Turkey. and Thanks-giving	Turkey is a great low-fat meat but the rest of the celebration dishes are not that fast-friendly, so I'd use the flexibility of this diet to eat what you like on the holiday itself, and then cut back later. It's a Feast Day, after all.	

U is for Ugli fruit	I've never had one. Apparently it's a bit like a grapefruit.	½ fruit = 45
V is for Vinegar	Vinegar is under-rated. In the UK, we love the strong malty sort on chips – so unlikely to feature in a Fast Day. But the world of vinegar includes fruit vinegars, sherry, cider, red and white wine and even champagne: these are virtually calorie free. As a dressing the milder ones can work on their own, without oil, and balsamic – which does contain more calories – is fab on cooked veg as well as salad. Sweet and sour, yummy! Plus apparently it has lots of medicinal benefits including positive effects on blood pressure, cholesterol and diabetes/insulin sensitivity (bit.ly/Ssvdcg)	1 teaspoon balsamic = 12-16 1 teaspoon white wine vinegar = 1!
W is for Watercress	Another one of those ingredients often quoted as a super-food because of its high levels of Vitamin C and other nutrients – it was recommended in the 16th century as a treatment for scurvy. It makes a nutritious salad or soup ingredient, and scientists are investigating cancer-fighting properties, too.	100g = 11g

X is for Xmas	As with Thanksgiving, the treats like mince pies and Christmas pud won't help with Fasts. But this diet is ideal for any kind of celebration - you can feel virtuous by simply fasting two days over the festive period, which might be a relief after so much rich food. Remember, this is for life, not just for Christmas	
Y is for Yogurt	Remember the thin, unpleasant smelling diet yogurts of the eighties and nineties? Now you can get very palatable tasting ones at below 100 calories. On Fast Days, though, I often prefer to use normal yogurt, or even Greek yogurt, in very tiny doll's house portions.	Depends on brand!

Treats, Snacks and Eating Out

To Snack or not to Snack

The debate about 'grazing' or snacking is one we've touched on in the book, and generally many 5:2 Dieters do avoid eating between (small) meals on Fast Days. But there are times when you just fancy something NOW and then it makes sense to go for the lower-calorie options rather than choose something that will undo all the hard work...

Health food shops are a good source of nuts or trail mix, but do check the nutritional values. My favourite snack food ever – Thai Chilli Rice Crackers – look as though they should be super-healthy but most are very high calorie...

I'm a fan of UK company *Graze.com* which delivers snacks in a letter-box sized container, with four mini-packs of sweet and savoury snacks including nuts, dried fruit and even chocolate mixes. Some are healthier than others but opening the pack every week is like getting a little present. You can ask for a Light option and they usually offer the first boxes at half-price.

I tend to find I crave either something sweet or savoury, so here are some options for those moments when a mug of green tea won't do.

Savoury Snacks and Treats

Snack	Calories
Miso soup: most sachets of miso soup with tofu or sea vegetables	25-35
Air popped popcorn, 1 cup	31
Olives: 10 pitted green olives	42
Oatcake Plus 2 teaspoons (10g) Philadelphia Light Or 1 teaspoon (5g) Peanut Butter as a topping	35-50 15 30
Red Mini Babybel (UK) Light Babybel (UK)	61 40
10 almonds (1 almond is 7 calories – will fill you up for ages)	70
1 rasher of grilled bacon and a dollop of ketchup	87
17g pack of Quavers	88
Pack savoury Snack a Jacks	92-108
1 bag of ready salted French Fries (crisps)	97
25g bag of Twiglets	98
10 Pringles	100

Sweet Snacks and Treats

Snack	Calories
Sugar-free jellies	5-15
Options Hot Chocolates Belgian chocolate	40
Milky Way Mini	40
Jaffa cake	46
Small scoop of soft-scoop vanilla ice-cream	50-60
10g 85% dark chocolate	55
2 medium peaches	76
20 Cherries	80
1 McVitie's chocolate digestive	84
Thin slice of malt loaf	85
1 small banana	90
2 ginger biscuits	90
Solero ice-cream (Berry and Tropical flavours)	90
5 dried apricots	95
4 dates	96
2 Cadbury's Roses	100
1 meringue nest with 6 strawberries	100

Eating Out

I am veering into the department of the obvious here but I try *not* to eat out on Fast Days as it's really hard to make good choices, plus you have no real idea how many calories you're consuming. You will have read earlier on in my diary about Temptation-Gate, where I went out planning to have soup at my favourite cafe, only to find it's not served at weekends. So I plumped for Eggs Florentine, which was probably my entire daily allowance, but kept me full all day.

If you are out and about, make the choices you'd make for other diets - ask for bread to be taken off the table, or give it to your dining companion. Choose soups, ideally non-creamy, and salads, and ask for the dressing on the side. Lean fish or chicken with veggies is not exciting but will usually give you some control. If all else fails - if you want to give into temptation or suddenly have something to celebrate - then it's even simpler. Fast tomorrow instead!

Fast Day Meal Plans for all Tastes

You've got all the tools you need to plan your own Fast Days – but as an extra aid, I've outlined some daily meal plans, using these recipes and ready-made meals. Use them as the basis for your own meal planning if you find it useful... or go your own way! There's also a blank template for your own use.

Of course, men get an extra 100 calories on top of the 500 allowed for women – so I've added an extra Man's Ration to those days!

An asterisk after the dish means the recipe is in this book.

The Big Salad Lunch Day

This is one of my real meal days – a massive, delicious, no-holds-barred salad eaten outdoors with friends on a picnic. Slightly over in terms of calories, but plenty of protein and fat that kept me from getting hungry until next day.

Meal	Food	Calories
Breakfast		
Lunch	Garofalo - Bufala Mozzarella, 0.5 container (2.2 oz/60g.)	**174**
	Peppery Baby leaf Rocket Salad, 15 g	**3**
	Sweet fire Beetroot, 75 g	**30**
	Balsamic Vinegar of Modena, 5ml	**5**
	Avocados - Raw, 49 g	
	Wholemeal mini roll	**78**
	Marks and Spencer - Traditional Coleslaw, 40 g	**86**
		132
Dinner		
Snacks		
Total		**508**

Optional Man Ration: 125 ml of chenin blanc white wine (perfect with this picnic salad) = 110 calories

A Soupy Day on the Go

A day to prove you have two fairly filling meals and a snack – or two snacks if you're male!

Meal	Food	Calories
Breakfast	Black coffee	
Lunch	Leek and Potato soup with White bread croutons	**120** **79**
Dinner	Home-Made Green & White Super Soup* Chicken breast 100g Salsa Broccoli, 100g, steamed 60g mushrooms fried with no-cal oil spray then heated with 20g Philadelphia with Chives	**76** **100** **14** **32** **10** **32**
Snacks	1 sugar-free Raspberry jelly	**10**
Total		**473**

Optional Man Ration: 1 medium banana (90 cals) or small bag of Twiglets (98 cals)

Family Friendly Feast

For those days when you don't want to cook separate dishes for the family – or when you don't want anyone to notice you're on a diet. Simply eat the same dishes but serve extras (granola and lots of yogurt for breakfast, extra toast with butter and cheese for lunch, portion of pilau rice and chicken or prawns for dinner) to your family and they won't even notice...

Meal	Food	Calories
Breakfast	Fresh raspberries 20	20
	25g Greek style yogurt	34
Lunch	Toast (1 slice)	92
	Beans (200g)	144
Dinner	Mushroom Tom Yum Soup*	40
	Vegetable curry*	150
Snacks		
Total		**480**

Optional Man Ration: 1/3ʳᵈ portion of Tilda microwaved wholegrain pilau = 98 calories

Three Square (Ready) Meals

Three satisfying but easily prepared meals for when you have very little time!

Meal	Food	Calories
Breakfast	Quaker Oatmeal Perfect Portions Cinnamon Instant Oatmeal	**160**
Lunch	Campbell's Soup On the Go Chicken with Mini Noodles Soup	**70**
Dinner	Cafe Steamers Honey Glazed Turkey and Sweet Potatoes	**250**
Snacks		
Total		**480**

Optional Man Ration: 1 stoneground bread roll or slice bread 80-95 calories

The Big Breakfast

Enjoy a super-satisfying breakfast/brunch to keep you full all day!

Meal	Food	Calories
Breakfast	2 rashers lean unsmoked back bacon	106
	2 portobello mushrooms grilled	45
	with	40
	1 tsp. olive oil	24
	8 cherry tomatoes on	90
	the vine	122
	1 slice granary bread	
	1 free range pork sausage, 86% pork, grilled	75
	1 free range egg, poached	
Lunch		
Dinner		
Snacks		
Total		**502**

Optional Man Ration: 125ml freshly squeezed orange juice (63 cals), 100 grams mixed frozen berries (30 cals) – either whole, or blended together as a smoothie.

Celebration Time

If you plan it carefully, you can still go to the ball... of course, when you're eating out, calories are approximate but these are all safe bets!

Meal	Food	Calories
Breakfast		
Lunch	1 portion Spicy Indian Lentil & Tomato soup*	130
Dinner	7 cherry tomatoes,	21
	7 carrot sticks	35
	4 cucumber sticks	4
	2 tablespoons	23
	hummus	15
	2 tablespoons salsa	55
	1 grilled chicken wing	125
	2 pieces nigri salmon sushi	
Snacks	Cava, 125 ml/4.2 fl. oz.	94
Total		**502**

Optional Man Ration:

2 x grissini Italian breadsticks (40 cals), 1 tablespoon guacamole (25), 1 mini cocktail sausage (30) = 95

Blank Planning Template

Use to plan and then monitor your own Fast Days. Record your mood and thoughts as you progress – to help you work out what's the best balance for you.

There's a downloadable, printable version via my website, kate-harrison.com/5-2diet

Date:			
Meal	Food	Calories	Mood & comments
Breakfast			
Lunch			
Dinner			
Snacks & drinks			
	Total		

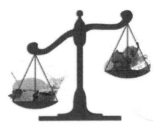

Resources, links and the last instalment of Kate's 5:2 diary

Further reading, a glossary and final words of encouragement!

Fasting and Healthy Eating Links

Don't forget that for readers of the print edition, I've put together a free downloadable list of all the links, to make it easier to follow up internet resources directly from your computer. It's available at kate-harrison.com/5-2diet and will save you a lot of typing!

The 'Horizon' Eat, Fast, Live Longer programme which inspired so many of us has a page at bbc.in/QPdsFC - it no longer shows the entire programme, but there are some clips. The programme was on YouTube but then was taken down because it breached copyright. Hopefully it will be repeated soon!

There's also an article by presenter Dr Mosley about his experiences on the BBC site (bbc.in/UuhPVU) as well as a similar one in the *Daily Telegraph* (bit.ly/11jCMol).

Diet Tools:

myfitnesspal.com has made this diet possible for me - and has lots of community forums and tools, plus a great app for Android and iPhone (free at the time of writing). The only drawback is that it does get quite cross with you for under-eating on your Fast Days as there's no option that I've found for telling it that you're only fasting/under-eating for a minority of the time.

Dr James Johnson's site – johnsonupdaydowndaydiet.com - has lots of interesting information on his alternate day fasting regime, though to get the full lowdown on his diet, you'd have to buy his book. It's not as flexible as the approach outlined here but it may work if you like to follow a stricter diet, and read more about the science.

Recipes

The 5:2 diet was featured in the *Daily Telegraph* and they had some tasty recipe suggestions (bit.ly/V637jU).
The excellent BBC Good Food recipes site allows you to specify courses, ingredients, preparation time and calorie counts – the user ratings are incredibly useful for tips and suggestions for improving the recipes too. You can also join so you can compile your own recipe 'binder'. As a first step this link has great dishes between 200-400 calories (bit.ly/SsvbkI)

The Tinned Tomatoes blog has featured a number of really tasty 5:2 suggestions (bit.ly/TsuLYD)

Forums:

The Mumsnet forum on 5:2 has become a treasure trove of brilliant advice and experiences – search for the different 5:2 and ADF threads in the weight loss forum (bit.ly/Tv3xUV) You definitely don't have to be a Mum to call on all that wisdom.

The Money Saving Expert Forum has a less active but still useful forum on the diet (bit.ly/ToawLX)

There are a number of 5:2 and fasting groups on Facebook - ours is called The 5:2 Diet and is very friendly. You can see the entries but need to join to post.

Diet Research and Discussion:

Mark's Daily Apple website has a focus on 'primal living' but there's a terrific amount of information on fasting, including summaries on the science (bit.ly/Uui9DP).

The Diabetes UK site has very clear information about GI values and diets as well as lots about the disease itself (bit.ly/Tv2B2Y) . There is also some information about religious fasting and how it affects diabetes, but as I've mentioned, anyone with a diabetes diagnosis should talk to a specialist before thinking about fasting for any reason.

Scientific and Medical research:

These two digests/reviews of research (bit.ly/113ykL3 and bit.ly/ShaV4h) are worth downloading to see the positives – as well as the doubts – about human and animal research. The latter also includes a look at religious fasting.

And this is a report on one ADF trial (bit.ly/QsGhGF). Science Daily has lots of interesting articles, written in fairly jargon-free language: start with this one bit.ly/QPeAsS and then follow the links.

Glossary:

5:2, 6:1 , 4:3   Different variations on fasting/calorie restriction – the second number is usually the number of days you follow restrictions in your diet.

ADF   Alternate Daily Fasting – cutting down or eating nothing every other day.

Bit.ly   Nothing to do with fasting, but a very useful way of shortening long web links – you can type these directly into your browser to find a recommended web page.

BMI   Body Mass Index – simple height/weight calculation used to gauge whether someone's weight may be putting their health at risk.

BMR   Basal Metabolic Rate – i.e. what your body needs in calorie terms for basic survival, without any activity other than basic functions

DCR	Daily Calorie Requirement – also known as Daily Calorie Need - an estimate of the number of calories you need that factors in your activity levels as well as age, height and weight.
Fast	Fast usually means eating nothing (and, in some religions, not drinking anything either). However, 5:2 dieters often use it as shorthand for days when they eat limited amounts.
Feast	Days when you eat normally. Also known as Feed Days.

Kate's 5:2 Diary Part Five: November 2012 and beyond...

The way to live - forever

Mood: hopeful, expectant, optimistic

Weight 30 November: 145 pounds: Total lost:16 pounds

BMI: 24.9 - in the healthy range, hooray!

Days on Diet: 113

So, after a very busy few weeks of working on my 5:2 book, I'm almost there. But although this is the end of this part of the process, it's not the end of the story.

Scientists are busy continuing research into intermittent fasting - while here at ground level, my weight loss continues. I've been 'dieting' now for almost four months and it gets easier, and easier. I'm looking forward to wearing my party dress and eating lots of Christmas food - I'll be fasting when I can but I also know that if I don't lose weight in December then there's still January and, well, the rest of my life.

As for resolutions… my number 1 goal on January 1 this year was to get back to a healthy weight. I know for certain it wouldn't have happened without 5:2 and I couldn't be more thrilled.

OK. I've failed at enough diets to know that you can never say never, but this new way of life is so different, and so satisfying, that I really do intend to stick to it.

I'll end by answering a few questions I've been asked over the last four months of living this way.

Have you considered giving up this diet?
Not once. With pretty much every other diet I've undertaken, I've already given up by month four. On this one, I might have the odd day when circumstances change - I fancy going out to celebrate something, or a friend calls out of the blue. But there's no beating myself up - I simply switch the Fast Day to tomorrow. This isn't all or nothing - it's about a small but permanent change.

Have you got a target weight in mind?
I'd like to be a tad under ten stone.
Because it's nice to be able to say nine
stone something. This would give me a BMI
of just under 24 - I could go lower, but
I'm naturally curvy (another way of saying,
I've got a big chest!) and when I got to
nine stone low-carbing, I was probably too
thin.

Will you abandon 5:2 once you reach the target?
No. I like the idea of reducing to a fast
one day a week, as a kind of 'check in' on
portion size and for the health benefits.
I'll also keep weighing myself once a week,
I think, because it's a good way to avoid
the weight 'creeping' back on.

Is this just another craze - see also Atkin's, Cabbage Soup Diet, the F-Plan?
My opinion - shared by many others - is
that this is different. It's not about
cutting out entire food groups, or eating
strange foods dreamed up by the diet
industry. For me, it's about people who are

overwhelmed by choice and the availability of food being helped to make better decisions. The appetite element, the flexibility, the health benefits and the all-round sustainability of it make it different.

Plus, it's a 'craze' that happens to have been around a very, very long time - from the unavoidable and frankly scary fast/feast lifestyle of early man, to the instructions to fast contained in so many religions. A respite or retreat from excess is something that has worked for humanity for many centuries. In the twentieth century, those who could, turned their back on the feeling of hunger, but now I've rediscovered what appetite and food mean to me.

A sense of perspective

I'm writing this on the evening of a Fast Day when I've eaten only one main meal, with no hunger pangs or ill effects. It reminds me how lucky we are to be able to choose what and when we eat. Fasting has done much more than help me lose weight -

it's helped me regain control over my eating habits and make me look forward to my next meal as one of the pleasures of life.

I really hope you've been inspired by the stories of the fantastic dieters who shared their struggles and their successes. I'd like to thank them for their ideas, and for their invaluable input on the drafts of this book.

I'd love it if you could share your own experiences of this way of life by getting in touch via my website, or joining our Facebook Group which you can find by searching for The 5:2 Diet.

I intend to update this ebook as and when there are further developments, and would love to include your story or tips in future editions so do please email me via my website, kate-harrison.com/5-2 diet, or follow @the52diet on Twitter for tips, updates and further free downloads!

Finally, if you've enjoyed this book, or would like to recommend it to others, I'd be so grateful if you'd think about leaving a review.

In the meantime, keep feasting, keep fasting and keep enjoying life!

Kate x

kate-harrison.com/5-2diet

Made in the USA
Lexington, KY
10 March 2013